P9-DNQ-669

CRITICAL THINKING IN NURSING

A Practical Approach

SECOND EDITION

Rosalinda Alfaro-LeFevre, RN, MSN
President, Teaching Smart/Learning Easy
Stuart, Florida

W.B. SAUNDERS COMPANY
A Division of Harcourt Brace & Company
Philadelphia   London   Toronto   Montreal   Sydney   Tokyo

W.B. SAUNDERS COMPANY

A Division of Harcourt Brace & Company

The Curtis Center
Independence Square West
Philadelphia, Pennsylvania 19106

Library of Congress Cataloging-in-Publication Data
Alfaro-LeFevre, Rosalinda.
Critical thinking in nursing : a practical approach / Rosalinda
Alfaro-LeFevre. — 2nd ed.
p.   cm.
Includes bibliographical references and index.
ISBN 0-7216-8277-4
1. Nursing.   2. Critical thinking.   I. Title.
[DNLM: 1. Decision Making nurses' instruction.   2. Nursing
Process.   WY 100 A385c 1999]
RT86.A34   1999
610.73—dc21
DNLM/DLC
98-47454

CRITICAL THINKING IN NURSING

ISBN 0-7216-8277-4

Printed in the United States of America

Last digit is the print number: 9   8   7   6   5   4   3   2   1

To

My Advisors,

here in the United States, in Canada, and throughout the world

Without your timely and insightful reviews and advice,
I couldn't have done it.

Advisors and Reviewers

United States

Ledjie Ballard, RN, MSN, CRNA

Independent Consultant for Perioperative Processes and Systems Management; Teaching Associate in Anesthesiology, University of Washington, Seattle, Washington

Margaret E. Briody, RN, MSN

University of Rochester School of Nursing, Rochester, New York

Kathleen K. Brogan, RN, MSN, MSHEd

Brogan and Associates, Performance Consultants, Philadelphia, Pennsylvania

Darlene D. Davis, RN, MA, BSN

Director, Nursing Development and Practice, Morton Plant Mease Health Care, Clearwater, Florida

Bonnie Eyler, RN, MSN, JD

Shareholder/Partner, Firm of Sonneborn Rutter Cooney Klingensmith & Eyler, West Palm Beach, Florida

Polly D. Fehler, RN, MSN, AS

Head, Department of Nursing, Tri-County Technical College, Pendleton, South Carolina

Nancy M. Flynn, RNC, MSN

Clinical Educator, Bryn Mawr Hospital, Bryn Mawr, Pennsylvania

Pauline M. Green, PhD, RN

Associate Professor, College of Pharmacy, Nursing, and Allied Health Sciences, Howard University, Washington, District of Columbia

Taylor D. Hartman, PhD

President, Color Code Communications, Inc., Midvale, Utah

Carol A. Hutton, EdD, ARNP

President, Hutton Associates/Management and Organizational Consultant; Adjunct Professor, School of Business and Entrepreneurship, Nova/Southeastern University, Fort Lauderdale, Florida

Joan M. Jenks, RN, PhD

Director, Undergraduate Programs, Thomas Jefferson University, Philadelphia, Pennsylvania

Sharon E. Johnson, RNC, MSN, CAN

Jefferson Home Health, Ardmore, Pennsylvania

Sandra Lynn Caddell Kirkland, RN, DNS

Union University, Germantown, Tennessee

Heidi P. Laird, MLA, BA

Programmer, Information Resources Support Center, SmithKline Beecham Clinical Laboratories, Collegeville, Pennsylvania

Steven M. LaPorte, MD

Jefferson Health System, Philadelphia, Pennsylvania

John Alexander Martin

Vice President, Sales and Marketing, MEDSCAPE, New York, New York

Carol R. Matz, RN, MSN

West Chester University, West Chester, Pennsylvania

Ann McCourt

Ormond Beach, Florida

Marycarol McGovern, RN, PhD

College of Nursing, Villanova University, Villanova, Pennsylvania

Judith C. Miller, RN, MS

President, Nursing Tutorial and Consulting Services, Clifton, Virginia

Kevin R. Miller

Professional Development Manager, Brigham Young University, Provo, Utah

Barbara A. Musinski, RN, C. BS

Masters Candidate, Education Leadership, Florida Atlantic University; Instructor, Practical Nursing Program, North Technical Education Center, Riviera Beach, Florida

John Nerness, MD, FACEP

Emergency Department, Indian River Memorial Hospital, Vero Beach, Florida

Terri Sue Patterson, RN, MSN, CRRN

Nursing Consultation Services LTD/LifeTrak LTD, Norristown, Pennsylvania

Linda Picklesimer, MSN, RN

Instructor, Nursing Department, Greenville Technical College, Greenville, South Carolina

James Riley

Health Information Services, National Data Corporation, Atlanta, Georgia

Mary Ellen Santucci, RN, MSN, CRRN

Thomas Jefferson University, Philadelphia, Pennsylvania

Linda J. Scheetz, RN, EdD, CS, CEN

Chairperson and Professor, Division of Nursing, Mount Saint Mary College, Newburgh, New York

Jean L. Smith, RN, BSN

Paoli Memorial Hospital, Paoli, Pennsylvania

Maria Eleni Sophocles, MD

Attending Physician, Department of Obstetrics and Gynecology, Overlook Hospital, Summit, New Jersey

Susanne N. Suchy, RN, MSN, AOCN

Instructor, Henry Ford Community College, Dearborn, Michigan; CNS/Case Manager Oncology Patient Services, Barbara Ann Karmanos Cancer Institute at Harper Hospital, Detroit, Michigan

Carol Taylor, RN, PhD, CSFN

Georgetown University, Washington, District of Columbia

Marcella R. Thompson, CSP, COHN-S

Safety Engineer, Cherry Semiconductor Corporation, East Greenwich, Rhode Island

Sylvia Anderson Whiting, PhD, RN, CS

Professor of Nursing and Researcher, South Carolina State University, Orangeburg, South Carolina

Zane Robinson Wolf, RN, PhD, FAAN

La Salle University School of Nursing, Phialdelphia, Pennsylvania

Toni C. Wortham, RN, MSN

Professor, Madisonville Community College, Madisonville, Kentucky

International

Cecile Boisvert, RN, MScN

Consultant-Educator, Group of Research and Education for Health Professionals, Saint-Aubin; Lecturer, University of Paris, Paris, France

Sheila J. Cameron, RN, EdD

Professor, School of Nursing, and Executive Dean, College of Graduate Studies and Research, University of Windsor, Windsor, Ontario, Canada

Professor Dame June Clark

Professor of Community Nursing, University of Wales Swansea, Wales, United Kingdom

Judy E. Boychuk Duchscher, RN, BSN, FCCM, MN

Nursing Faculty, Nursing Education Program of Saskatchewan, Kelsey Campus, Saskatoon, Saskatchewan, Canada

Aiko Emoto, RN, MPH

Professor, Saniku Gakuin College, Japan

Ana M. Gimenez

Nursing Professor, Puerta de Hierro School of Nursing, Universidad Autonoma de Madrid, Madrid, Spain

Dr Megan-Jane Johnstone

Professor of Nursing, Department of Nursing Inquiry, Practice, and Management and Faculty of Biomedical and Health Sciences and Nursing, RMIT University, Bundoora, Victoria, Australia

Maria Teresa Luis

Enfermera, Licenciada en Antropologia, Profesora de Enfermeria Medico-Quirsurgica, Escuela de Enfermeria, Universidad de Barcelona, Barcelona, Spain

Judith Anne Manning, RN, RM, MA (Women's Studies), FRCNA

Lecturer, Faculty of Nursing, University of South Australia, Adelaide, Australia

Jeanne Liliane Marlene Michel, RN, BNS

Lecturer at the Department of Nursing, Federal University of Sao Paulo, Sao Paulo, Brazil

N.E. Oud, RN, Dipl.N.Adm., MNSc

Consultant and Trainer, Broens & Oud, Partnership for Consult and Training, The Netherlands

Dickon Weir-Hughes, RN, MA, BScN

Chief Nurse and Director of Patient Services, The Royal Marsden Hospitals, London and Surrey, England

Preface

WHAT'S PRACTICAL ABOUT THIS APPROACH?

Like the first edition, this book encourages you to identify strategies to think critically in your *own* way. With the help of examples, stories, illustrations, and practice exercises, you use critical thinking as you're learning about critical thinking.

- **Chapters 1 and 2** provide the foundation for learning how to think critically in various situations. The focus here is mainly on examining critical thinking in our daily lives, with some reference to nursing situations. Chapter 1 looks at *what* critical thinking is. Chapter 2 addresses *how* to think critically.
- **Chapters 3 and 4** focus specifically on critical thinking in the context of *nursing*.
- **Chapter 5** provides opportunities to practice essential critical thinking skills using case scenarios based on real nursing experiences.
- **Chapter 6** provides strategies and exercises for mastering abilities related to workplace skills as described in *Learning a Living: A Blueprint for High Performance, a SCANS* Report for America 2000.* This chapter covers skills like communicating

---

*Secretary's Commission on Achieving Necessary Skills (SCANS), Washington, DC. U.S. Department of Labor, 1992

bad news, working in teams, managing conflict, and dealing with mistakes and complaints.

WHAT'S NEW IN THIS EDITION

Here's what's new:

1. **Completely revised and updated.** Reflects current changes in health care delivery
   - More on multidisciplinary practice and use of computers and critical paths.
   - Strong focus on outcome-driven, evidence-based care.
   - Addresses the shift from a model of *diagnose and treat* to *predict, prevent, and manage.*
2. **More information from leaders in critical thinking.** Addresses both education and practice perspectives.
3. **Completely new chapter (Chapter 6).** Helps you master abilities related to common workplace skills as addressed above.
4. **Broad application.** Input from the multidisciplinary domestic and international advisory board has been included in the final manuscript.
5. **A new kind of HMO.** In accordance with my belief that humor sends strong messages and is good for the soul, I'm pleased to annouce the publication of two clips from my comic strip, *HMO (Help Me Out).* This comic addresses the funny and ridiculous things that happen to care-

givers and receivers. If you'd like to share a story involving the care of a patient, friend, family member, or pet, please contact me at the address given at the end of this preface.

WHAT'S THE SAME ABOUT THIS EDITION

The following is retained from the first edition:

1. **User friendly.** Great pains have been taken to include design elements that motivate you to want to read and allow you to use your own way of mastering content (see page xi, The Best Way to Read This Book).
2. **Concise and applied.** Provides lots of useful information and strategies in a concise format. Includes theory, strategies, and critical thinking and practice exercises.
3. **Motivational style.** The writing style is informal, interactive, and designed to make you feel like you're "right there" having a personal discussion. The scenarios and exercises, based on real experience, are designed to simulate clinical nursing situations.*
4. **Solid content.** Comprehensive coverage on critical thinking in context of clinical practice and every day life.

A WORD ABOUT "PATIENT/CLIENT" AND "HE/SHE"

Whenever possible, a fictitious name, or "someone," "person," "consumer," or "individual" is used (instead of "patient" or "client") to help us keep in mind that each patient or client is a *person* who has unique needs, values, perceptions, and motivations. *He* and *she* are used interchangeably to avoid the awkwardness of using "he or she" all the time.

INSTRUCTORS' GUIDE AVAILABLE

To free faculty to direct creative energies toward *refining and improving* teaching strategies, rather than starting from scratch, an instructor's guide is available.

PLEASE TELL US WHAT YOU THINK

We want to hear your struggles and concerns. Whether you're a student or faculty member, if you're having a problem with something, it's likely others are too. Your problems are our opportunities to learn, improve, and help others with the same concerns. Please let us know what you think. Address comments to me or to Thomas Eoyang, Vice President and Editor-in-Chief, Nursing Books, W.B. Saunders Company, The Curtis Center, Independence Square West, Philadelphia, PA 19106.

Rosalinda Alfaro-LeFevre, RN, MSN
6161 SE Landing Way #9
Stuart, Florida 34997
Email: r-alfaro@juno.com

---

*Names and some facts are changed to provide anonymity.

The Best Way to Read This Book

THE BEST WAY TO READ THIS BOOK IS HOWEVER YOU CHOOSE TO READ IT

1. For those of you who like the traditional approach, read it from beginning to end. You'll enjoy the narrative, logical approach and numerous scenarios and examples designed to help you understand and *remember* content.
2. For those of you who like to use your own unique approach—for example, the *back to front* approach (read summaries before text), the *skip around to the stuff that looks interesting* approach, or the *read the stuff that will be on the test first* approach—here are some of the features that help you focus on what's most important.

PRECEDING EACH CHAPTER

- **This Chapter at a Glance:** Allows you to scan major headings.
- **Prechapter Self-Test and Learning Outcomes:** help you decide how to focus your thinking about content and where to spend most of your time.
- **Abstract:** Gives the big picture of what the chapter is all about.

FOLLOWING EACH CHAPTER

- **Key Points:** Provide a detailed summary of the most important content.

- **Critical Thinking Exercises and Practice Exercises:** Direct you to *use* content, helping you clarify understanding and move information into long-term memory.

OTHER FEATURES YOU NEED TO KNOW ABOUT

- **Glossary:** Provides definitions of key terms. If you don't understand words, look them up, or you may miss major points.
- **Critical Moments:** Give simple strategies that can make a BIG difference in improving your efficiency and productivity.
- **Other Perspectives:** Offer interesting (and sometimes amusing) points of view encountered during manuscript preparation.
- **Response Key:** Example responses for Critical Thinking Exercises and Practice Exercises are provided to help you evaluate your responses. This is called a *response key,* rather than an *answer key,* to avoid implying that there's *only one right answer* to each question. In many cases, a variety of responses are acceptable (great minds don't always think alike). The main point of the exercises isn't necessarily to come up with the right responses: Rather, the point is to get in touch with the thinking that led you to your response, and to be able to evaluate and correct your thinking as needed.

READING EFFICIENTLY

However you choose to read, keep in mind the following steps, which provide an organized and efficient way to master content.

- **Survey:** Scan the abstract, major headings, tables, and illustrations.
- **Question:** Turn major headings into questions.
- **Read:** Read, taking notes and answering your questions.
- **Review, Recite, and Re-read:** Review the chapter (or your notes), reciting key content out loud. Then ask yourself, "What's still not clear here?" Read the sections you don't understand again; raise questions to ask in class or discuss with your peers.

Acknowledgments

I want to thank my husband, Jim, for his love, support, and sense of humor and fun. I also want to thank the rest of my family and the following people for their belief in me and their contribution to my personal and professional growth:

Grace and Frank Nola, Emily Barrosse, Marty Kenney, Heidi Laird, Ledjie Ballard, Terri Patterson, Nancy Flynn, Carol Taylor, Connie Sechrist, Becky Resh, Diane Verity, Annette Sophocles, Barbara Cohen, Patti Cleary, Carol Hutton, Bonnie Eyler, Lynda Carpenito, Nat and Louise Rochester, Charlie and Nancy Lindsay, Bill and Mary Jo Boyer, John Payne, the Villanova College of Nursing Faculty, and the past and present staff nurses of Paoli Memorial Hospital.

My special thanks go to the following people at W.B. Saunders: Thomas Eoyang, Vice President and Editor-in-Chief, Nursing Books, for his belief in this project, consistent support, and high standards; Amelia Cullinan, Editorial Assistant, for her patience and attention to detail; John Cooke, Executive Vice President, Production Services; Judy Schmitt, designer; Mary Espenschied, copy editor; Joan Sinclair, Production Manager; and the sales and marketing staff for their crucial role in making this book successful.

Rosalinda Alfaro-LeFevre

Assumptions and Promises

Before I began to write this book, I made some assumptions:

- You want to learn.
- Your time is valuable, and you don't want to waste it.
- You like to learn the most important things first.
- You learn better when you're motivated, know why information is relevant, and choose your own way of learning.
- It's inappropriate for *me* to tell *you* how to think.
- You feel a sense of accomplishment when you master knowledge and skills that help you be more independent.

Because of these assumptions, I promise to:

- Let you know what's most important.
- Use lots of examples and present information in a usable way.
- Provide the "reasons behind the rules."
- Encourage you to *choose* what works for *you*.
- Help you gain or refine the skills required to be a better thinker, independent learner, and more effective nurse.

Introduction: More Than a TV Show

Nurses regularly encounter dramas that most people see only on television. Think about the collective voice of some of our colleagues:

 OTHER PERSPECTIVES

Too Much at Stake

"As health care professionals, we hold human health and well-being in our hands. Who we choose to be on any given day may literally determine how someone is born, lives, or dies. Too much is at stake for us to treat this responsibility lightly."

—*Carol Taylor, RN, MSN, PhD, Author and Healthcare Ethicist*

People in Dangerous Territory

"[The] hospital is a dangerous place. It's the unusual patient who escapes without at least one scar: a phlebitis from an intravenous line, a miserable morning undergoing a poorly thought out barium enema, anxiety over the when and why of the next blood drawing, the emptiness of disenfranchisement from decisions affecting his own integrity and sanity. One must therefore be sure the hospitalized patient belongs in the hospital; as soon as the patient can function at home safely and comfortably, let him go."*

—*Mark Fishman, MD, Physician and Author*

Heavy Hands

"Occasionally we hold a person's life in our hands; almost always his dignity."

—*Leah L. Curtin, MS, MA, ScD(h), FAAN, Editor and Publisher,* Curtain Calls

As you can see from the preceding quotes, nurses hold great power over the human experience. Your ability to think well directly impacts on the care you give. As you read this book, I ask you to stretch your mind and think about new ways to acquire the intellectual skills needed to meet the challenges of health care delivery in a rapidly changing world. You owe it to your patients and to yourself. You're a real nurse. You don't play one on TV.

---

*Fishman, M., Hoffman, A., Klaus, R., and Thaler, M. (1991). *Medicine* (p. v). Philadelphia: J.B. Lippincott.

Contents

3 CRITICAL THINKING IN NURSING: AN OVERVIEW 56

6 APPLIED CRITICAL THINKING: MASTERING COMMON WORKPLACE SKILLS 186

RESPONSE KEY 238

CRITICAL THINKING
IN NURSING

1

Overview: What Is Critical Thinking and Why Is It Important?

This chapter at a glance . . .

Read the Learning Outcomes listed below and decide whether you can readily achieve each one. If you can, you don't need to read this chapter and can go on to Chapter 2. Don't be concerned if you can't achieve any of the outcomes at this time. We'll come back to these outcomes later in the chapter, in Critical Thinking Exercises.

Suggestion: *Reading with a purpose* is a key strategy that triggers your brain to get involved in what you're reading, carefully evaluating the material and making decisions about what's important and how the material might be used. Mark your book or take notes when you encounter information that will help you achieve the objectives.

LEARNING OUTCOMES

After studying this chapter, you should be able to:

- Describe critical thinking using your own words, based on a commonly seen description of critical thinking.

- Explain the difference between thinking and critical thinking.

- Give at least three reasons why critical thinking is essential for nurses.

- Explain the relationship between outcomes (results) and critical thinking.

- Describe five critical thinking characteristics, traits, or dispositions you'd like to develop or improve.

- Address how critical thinking is similar to and different from problem solving.

- Identify four principles of the scientific method that are evident in critical thinking.

ABSTRACT

This chapter focuses on the big picture of critical thinking. It begins by addressing why critical thinking is essential and how this book helps improve thinking skills. It then takes a closer look at critical thinking, asking you to consider questions like, What's the difference between thinking and critical thinking? How is critical thinking commonly described? What are the characteristics, traits, and dispositions of critical thinkers? and What's familiar and what's new about critical thinking?

WHY FOCUS ON CRITICAL THINKING?

To address the question, Why focus on critical thinking? I like to start with another question: Have you noticed that nothing seems simple anymore—that as we improve and progress, life only seems to get more complicated? Think about some examples:

- People live longer with more chronic and complex problems providing new challenges.
- Computers give us instant access to vast knowledge stores, making it hard to find what it is *we* need.
- In communities, schools, and especially in the workplace, we're all expected to accept more responsibilities, work with diverse teams, and make more independent judgments and decisions (see Table 1–1 and Box 1–1).

If we want to survive—better yet, *thrive*—we must be able to think critically. We must know how to clearly and quickly focus our thinking in such a way that it gets the results we want, whether it be helping patients reach cost-effective outcomes, resolving conflicts with peers, or mastering new knowledge and skills.

In nursing, we have some additional reasons for teaching and learning about critical thinking:

1. Nurses are frequently involved in complex situations that increase responsibilities. We must view ourselves as knowledge workers—thinkers, not just doers.
2. Critical thinking is the key to resolving problems. Nurses who don't think critically become *part* of the problem.

TABLE 1–1	Changing Workplace

TODAY'S WORKPLACE	OLD WORKPLACE
Multiskilled workers who: • Take ownership and responsibility • Cross barriers once clearly defined • Engage in group problem solving	Narrow job descriptions with isolated performance with narrow caregiver roles
Innovation (many ways) *unless* research shows one approach consistently works better than another (evidenced-based care)	One best way to do things (often yours; not much evidence to support yours is best)
Decentralization and self-directed work groups where all workers are responsible for productivity and maintaining a positive organizational image	Centralized management with little room for self-direction

BOX 1–1	Workplace Skills*

To succeed in the workplace and as learners, you must know how to:

- **Use** resources: allocate time, money, materials, space, and human resources.
- **Establish** positive interpersonal relationships: work on teams, teach others, lead, negotiate, and work well with culturally diverse individuals.
- **Acquire** and evaluate information: organize and maintain files, interpret and communicate, and use computers to process information.
- **Assess** social, organizational, and technological systems: monitor and correct performance and design or improve systems.
- **Use** technology: select equipment and tools, apply technology to tasks, maintain and troubleshoot equipment.

Accomplishing the above requires you to have:

- **Basic skills:** reading, writing, mathematics, speaking, and listening.
- **Thinking skills:** knowing how to learn, reason, think creatively, generate and evaluate ideas, see things in the mind's eye, make decisions, and solve problems.
- **Personal qualities:** responsibility, self-esteem, self-confidence, self-management, sociability, and integrity.

*Adapted from The Secretary's Commission on Achieving Necessary Skills [SCANS], The U.S. Department of Labor. (1992). *Learning a living: A blueprint for high performance, a SCANS report for America 2000* (p. xiv). Washington, D.C.: The Author.

3. Critical thinking is essential to passing the National Council Licensure Examination (NCLEX).
4. Accreditation visitors to both schools and health care facilities look for evidence of critical thinking ability.

HOW DOES THIS BOOK HELP DEVELOP THINKING SKILLS?

This book is based on the belief that thinking is just like any other skill (music, art, athletics), that we each have our own styles and innate or learned capabilities. And we can all improve by gaining insight, acquiring instruction and feedback, and consciously practicing to improve.

This book is organized to encourage you to use your own thinking as a major tool for learning:

- **This chapter and Chapter 2** provide the foundation for learning how to think critically in various situations. The focus here is mainly on examining critical thinking in our daily lives with some reference to nursing situations. This chapter looks at *what* critical thinking is. Chapter 2 addresses *how* to think critically.
- **Chapters 3 and 4** focus specifically on critical thinking in the context of *nursing*.
- **Chapter 5** provides opportunities to practice essential critical thinking skills using case scenarios based on real nursing experiences.
- **Chapter 6** provides strategies and exercises for mastering abilities related to workplace skills as described in *Learning a Living: A Blueprint for High Performance, a SCANS Report for America 2000.*[1] This chapter covers skills like communicating bad news, working in teams, managing conflict, and dealing with mistakes and complaints.

WHAT'S THE DIFFERENCE BETWEEN THINKING AND CRITICAL THINKING?

Consider the following scenarios:

Scenario One

It's Tuesday. You're driving down the highway and these thoughts are going through your mind: "I'll sure be glad when this week is over. I have so much to do . . . anatomy test on Wednesday . . . paper due on Thursday . . . work, tonight. . . . I really wanted to get a hair cut. . . . Do I really have to shop tomorrow? . . . Gee, what an interesting looking man that is on the corner. . . . I'm starving . . . what can I eat?"

Scenario Two

It's Wednesday and you're taking the anatomy test. You're completely surprised by one of the questions. Your stomach becomes knotted and you think, "I don't have a clue what this answer is. . . . I can't believe I don't know this. . . . I studied hard, but I don't remember this. . . . I can't believe it. . . . When did we talk about this? . . . We never covered this, did we? . . . I've got to get myself together and think . . . hmmm . . . think, think, think. If I could only think. . . . Ten more minutes. . . . I've got to get thinking. . . . I hate when this happens."

Scenario Three

It's Friday. You've had a bad week. The anatomy test was terrible. You were stressed out at work because you were worried about your paper. You finished your paper in a last-minute rush. You look ahead and feel overwhelmed with assignments and commitments. You think to yourself, "I've got to get organized." You sit down, figure out your most important goals, and develop a sensible plan to reach them. Staying focused on the most important priorities, you develop a daily and weekly schedule designed to help you stay on track. You also make an appointment to talk with your advisor about resources that may be able to help you with specific problems (e.g., where you can get help with test-taking skills).

Scenario One shows aimless thinking with ideas and images drifting through your head. **Scenario Two** shows attempts to begin thinking to answer the test question, but your mind is stuck on negative thoughts that get you nowhere. **Scenario Three** shows focused, deliberate thought. You recognize that your brain is overwhelmed with all that is going on; you take control, get organized, and take steps to make the most of your brainpower. You begin to think critically.

So what's the difference between thinking and critical thinking? The key difference is control and purpose. Thinking is basically any mental activity—it can be aimless and uncontrolled. On the other hand, critical thinking is controlled and purposeful and focuses on using *well-reasoned* strategies to achieve desired results.

CRITICAL THINKING: SOME DIFFERENT DESCRIPTIONS

Because critical thinking is a complex activity that can be described in more than one way, there's no one *right* definition. Many authors (including myself) develop their own descriptions to complement and clarify someone else's (which is, by the way, a good example of thinking critically—critical thinking requires you to "personalize" information—to analyze it and decide what it means to you rather than simply memorizing words).

Consider the following synonym and commonly seen descriptions. Don't try to memorize them. Just think about which one makes most sense to you.

A Synonym

If you ever hear, "Give me one word that explains critical thinking," a good word to offer is *reasoning*. If you were in elementary school today, you'd be learning the 4 Rs instead of three: reading, 'riting, 'rithmetic, and *reasoning*. Beginning in kindergarten, children are learning the *how to's* of effective reasoning (e.g., how to gain insight to solve problems and make wise decisions). This fourth R continues to be stressed throughout the primary and secondary schools. Tomorrow's world will be full of people who learned reasoning skills, or critical thinking skills, from a very early age.

Now you have a synonym for critical thinking—*reasoning*. Because reasoning is a highly individualized, complex activity that involves *distinct ideas, emotions, and perceptions*, let's move on to a more substantial discussion.

Common Descriptions of Critical Thinking

Here are some commonly seen descriptions of critical thinking:

- "Knowing how to learn, reason, think creatively, generate and evaluate ideas, see things in the mind's eye, make decisions and solve problems."[1]
- "Reasonable, reflective thinking that focuses on what to believe or do."[2]
- "The art of thinking about your thinking, while you're thinking, to make it better, more clear, accurate, and defensible."[3]

- "Purposeful and goal-directed thinking."[4]
- "The process of purposeful, self-regulatory judgment . . . the cognitive engine that drives problem-solving and decision-making."[5]

What Is Critical Thinking in Nursing?

In search of a useful definition for describing nursing's critical thinking, I reviewed the literature, considered today's nursing roles, and developed the following description.

Critical thinking in nursing:
- Entails purposeful, outcome-directed (results-oriented) thinking.
- Is driven by patient, family, and community needs.
- Is based on principles of nursing process and scientific method.
- Requires knowledge, skills, and experience.
- Is guided by professional standards and ethics codes.
- Requires strategies that maximize human potential (e.g., using individual strengths) and compensate for problems created by human nature (e.g., the powerful influence of personal perspectives, values, and beliefs).
- Is constantly reevaluating, self-correcting, and striving to improve.

We'll look at what critical thinking in nursing entails in depth in Chapters 3 and 4. For now, keep in mind the following rule:

▨ **Rule:** Critical thinking is purposeful and outcome focused (results oriented). To think critically in any situation, you must be clear about your purpose: What exactly are the results you want?

WHAT DO CRITICAL THINKERS LOOK LIKE?

When we ask, What do critical thinkers look like? we mean, What characteristics do we see in someone who thinks critically? Consider the following description:

The ideal critical thinker is habitually inquisitive, self-informed, trustful of reason, open-minded, flexible, fair-minded in evaluation, honest in facing personal biases, prudent in making judgments, willing to reconsider, clear about issues, orderly in complex matters, diligent in seeking relevant information, reasonable in selection of criteria, focused in inquiry, and persistent in seeking results which are as precise as the subject and the circumstances of inquiry permit.[6]

Now you have a somewhat lengthy description of what the ideal critical thinker looks like. Let's look at the characteristics or attitudes of critical thinkers.

Characteristics (Attitudes) of Critical Thinkers

Knowing the characteristics frequently seen in those who think critically helps you get a holistic view of what critical thinking is: If you consider the characteristics, or attitudes, of those who consistently demonstrate critical thinking, you have an overall picture of what it takes to think critically. Look at Box 1–2, which provides a list of characteristics of critical thinkers. Compare yourself with each quality described, putting a "W" next to the ones you feel you've developed *well* and an "I" next to those you'd like to *improve*. Keep in mind that some of the best minds are tempted to mark that they'd like to improve almost all their characteristics (because they believe there's always room for improvement). If you aren't *tempted* to put at least a few "I's," it's likely that you need to give this activity more thought.

Intellectual Traits and Dispositions

Richard Paul, Director of The Center for Critical Thinking, and researchers Norreen and Peter Facione offer another way to look at the characteristics displayed by critical thinkers. Paul addresses the need to develop what he calls "intellectual traits of the mind."[3] The Faciones identify seven critical thinking dispositions—seven habits of the mind—that are evident in those who think critically.[5,7,8] Some of Paul's intellectual traits and the Faciones' critical thinking dispositions are listed below.

Paul's Intellectual Traits[3]
- **Intellectual humility:** Willingness to admit what you don't know.
- **Intellectual integrity:** Continual evaluation of your own thinking, holding yourself to the same standards you hold others, and willingness to admit when your thinking may be flawed.

| **BOX 1–2** | **Characteristics (Attitudes) of Critical Thinkers** |

Critical thinkers are:

- **Active thinkers,** maintaining a questioning attitude and double-checking both the reliability of the information and their own interpretation of it.
- **Fair-minded,** keenly aware of the powerful influence of their own perceptions, values, and beliefs but seeking to treat all viewpoints alike.
- **Persistant** and willing to exert a conscious effort to work in a planful manner, gathering information, checking for accuracy, and *persevering,* even when solutions aren't obvious or require several steps.
- **Good communicators,** realizing that *mutual exchange of ideas* is essential to understanding the facts and finding the best solutions.
- **Open-minded,** willing to consider other perspectives and suspending judgment until all the evidence is weighed.
- **Empathetic,** putting their own feelings aside and consciously imagining themselves in the place of others in order to genuinely understand them.
- **Independent thinkers,** striving to make their own judgments and decisions, rather than depending on others to do it for them.
- **Curious and insightful,** questioning deeply and interested in understanding underlying thoughts and feelings.
- **Humble,** being concerned about maintaining awareness of their own biases and limitations and being aware that no one, including themselves, knows everything.
- **Honest with themselves and others,** admitting when their conclusions may be flawed or require more thought.
- **Proactive,** instead of *reactive,* anticipating problems and acting *before* they occur.
- **Organized and systematic in their approach** to examining information, solving problems, and making decisions.
- **Flexible,** able to explore and imagine alternatives and change approaches and priorities as needed.
- **Cognizant of rules of logic,** recognizing the role of intuition but seeking evidence and weighing risks and benefits before acting.
- **Realistic,** acknowledging that we don't live in a perfect world and that the best answers aren't always the perfect answers.
- **Team players,** willing to collaborate to work toward common goals.
- **Creative and committed to excellence,** continually evaluating, seeking clarity and accuracy, and looking for ways to improve how things get done.

TABLE 1–2	Critical Thinking: What It Is and What It's Not	
CRITICAL THINKING	**NOT CRITICAL THINKING**	**EXAMPLE OF CRITICAL THINKING**
Criticism for the sake of improvement, new ideas, and doing things in the best interest of the key players involved	Criticism for the sake of attacking without being able to suggest new ideas or alternatives; critical for the sake of having it your way	Determining key players, then looking for flaws in the way something is done and figuring out better ways to achieve the same outcomes
Inquisitive about intent, facts, and reasons behind ideas or actions; thought and knowledge oriented	Unconcerned about motives, facts, and reasons behind ideas or actions; task oriented rather than thought oriented	Raising vital questions to better understand what happened, why it happened, and what was trying to be accomplished when it happened
Sensitive to the powerful influence of emotions but focused on making decisions based on facts and what's morally and ethically the right thing to do	Emotion driven; making decisions based on feelings rather than on consideration of what's the right thing to do	Finding out how someone feels about something, then moving on to discuss what's morally and ethically right
Thinking independently unless dealing with complex issues or a situation too risky to approach with limited knowledge	Continually looking to others for answers	Thinking things through independently; seeking help and multidisciplinary approaches as indicated

- **Intellectual courage:** Awareness of the need to face and fairly address ideas, beliefs, or viewpoints to which you have negative feelings and to which you haven't given serious hearing.
- **Intellectual empathy:** A conscious effort to understand others by putting your own feelings aside and imagining yourself in their place.

Faciones' Critical Thinking (CT) Dispositions[8]

1. "**Truthseeking:** A courageous desire for the best knowledge, even if such knowledge fails to support or undermines one's preconceptions, beliefs or self-interest.
2. "**Open-Mindedness:** Tolerance to divergent views, self-monitoring for possible bias.
3. "**Analyticity:** Demanding the application of reason and evidence, alert to problematic situations, inclined to anticipate consequences.

4. "**Systematicity:** Valuing organization, focus and diligence to approach problems of all levels of complexity.
5. "**CT Self-Confidence:** Trusting of one's own reasoning skills and seeing oneself as a good thinker.
6. "**Inquisitiveness:** Curious and eager to acquire knowledge and learn explanations even when the applications of the knowledge are not immediately apparent.
7. "**Maturity:** Prudence in making, suspending, or revising judgment. An awareness that multiple solutions can be acceptable. An appreciation of the need to reach closure even in the absence of complete knowledge."[8]

Table 1–2 gives some examples of what critical thinking is and what it's not.

■ **Want to know more?** Appendix A, page 250, summarizes what some experts say about critical thinking and tells you how to contact some national critical thinking resources.

REFLECTION AND INSIGHT ("HEMMING AND HAWING" AND AHA!)

Once I asked a student how she went about answering test questions. She replied, "usually I read the question, then I hem and haw about what's being asked and what's the best response." Critical thinking requires reasonable, reflective thinking—it may require you to "hem and haw."

Another expression that describes critical thinking is aha! We say aha! when we suddenly realize something or have our suspicions confirmed. We say aha! when we connect with something that was in the back of our minds but never put into words—when our gut feelings tell us something is right. The aha! experience is suddenly gaining awareness or insight into something that we have been trying to understand.

I hope that as you read this book you do a lot of "hemming and hawing" (reflecting) about what you read. If you're not sure about something or want to give it more thought, write a brief question in the margin or on a piece of paper to remind yourself to come back to it. Then discuss your thoughts with a teacher or someone else. You'll be surprised how much more you'll gain from your reading. Discussing key questions with others helps you clarify your thoughts, broaden your perspectives, and *understand* and *retain* what you read. I also hope you find ahas as you read. These moments of "light bulbs going off in your head" are energizing. They often bring you new ideas, build your confidence, and stimulate you to learn more.

CRITICAL MOMENT

Questions Please

Socrates learned more from questioning others than he did from reading books. Seek others' opinions and question deeply to gain understanding.

WHAT'S FAMILIAR AND WHAT'S NEW ABOUT CRITICAL THINKING

We understand something new best by comparing it with something we already know: How is it the same and how is it different? This section first addresses critical thinking concepts you're likely to find familiar; then it addresses concepts that are likely to be new.

What's Familiar

Problem Solving. In many ways, critical thinking is an upgraded version of the problem-solving method. It covers solving problems, but it acknowledges that having a problem-solving mentality isn't enough. Critical thinking also requires that you focus on improvement, asking questions like, What new knowledge and skills do I need? and How can we do this better?

Critical thinking may also be triggered by positive events as well as problems. For example, if you see something good happen, you should be thinking, *Hey! That's great! We need to see if we can make this happen more frequently (or for everybody).*

Analytical Thinking. Some people believe analytical thinking *is* critical thinking—and it's true, critical thinking requires analytical thinking. However, critical thinking involves more than analyzing. It involves focusing on results, considering how much time you have, and *drawing conclusions* about what you've analyzed. To think critically, you must avoid "analysis paralysis."

The Scientific Method and Nursing Process. There's a lot about critical thinking that's similar to principles of science, the scientific method, and nursing process. For example, critical thinking requires all of the following:

- **Observing.** Continuously observing and examining to collect data, check for changes, and gain understanding.
- **Classifying data.** Grouping related information in order to reveal relationships among the observed facts.
- **Drawing conclusions that follow logically.** If this is so, then. . . .
- **Conducting experiments.** Performing studies to examine hypotheses (suspicions) and identify ways to improve.
- **Testing hypotheses.** Determining whether the evidence that supports what we *believe* to be true *is* true.

What's New

Maximizing Human Potential. We're only just beginning to learn how to maximize the human potential to think critically. For example, as youngsters most of us were encouraged to memorize. However, few of us learned *how to memorize* in ways that promote comprehension and retention. We now know that memorizing a list of facts can be a dead end for our minds. It doesn't help us *understand* information, and it doesn't help us *remember it in the long term.* We're beginning to identify strategies like using visual centers of the brain and using preferred learning styles to maximize understanding and retention. We'll examine how to use these and other strategies in Chapter 4.

More Emphasis on the Need to Develop What-if Strategies. We now pay more attention to developing detailed approaches, policies, and procedures to cover what-if scenarios. For example, what do you do if you have to give someone bad news or what should you do when mistakes happen (see pages 192 to 194).

Interpersonal Skills and Group Thinking. Greater emphasis is being placed on the importance of mastering interpersonal skills and knowing how to facilitate group thinking. Today we must collaborate and facilitate "meetings of the minds" more than ever.

Box 1–3 gives an overview of additional things that are new about critical thinking. Figure 1–1 is a visual summary of questions that can help you evaluate your potential to think critically.

BOX 1-3	**What's New About Critical Thinking**

- Research findings suggesting that intelligence quotient (IQ) tests may not really measure IQ and that there are other focuses of intelligence (e.g., interpersonal intelligence) that influence our ability to think critically.
- The idea that thinking can and must be taught, that practicing thinking skills helps us be better thinkers.
- Information from the disciplines of neurology and neurosurgery suggesting that the brain is like a muscle: The more you use it, the more capable it becomes.
- The belief that personal interests, passions, and commitments, as well as a sense of esthetics (beauty), mystery, and wonder, play a crucial role in developing attitudes necessary for thinking.
- Increased concern about the *process* of reasoning: It's often as important to know *how* a conclusion or decision is made, as it is to know *what* the conclusion or decision is.
- Greater emphasis on understanding other perspectives and using several *different* perspectives (collaborate) to come to better conclusions. Great minds don't always think alike: Different viewpoints enhance our thinking.
- More acceptance of "There's more than one way" and "Sometimes there are no *right* answers" (each answer is correct in its own way).
- Increased acknowledgment that there are *useful mistakes* (occasional failure is the price of improvement) and that sharing mistakes is a responsible action that helps others avoid the same errors.
- More research on finding ways to "measure" how someone thinks.
- The identification of strategies that help us take advantage of how our brains work, including how to:
  - Get information into long-term memory
  - Form good habits of inquiry
  - Use both sides of our brains
  - Enhance creativity

SUMMARY

By now, you should have an idea of *what* critical thinking is and *why* it's important. To solidify your understanding, review the following Key Points and then complete the Critical Thinking Exercises that follow. Once you've done that, go on to Chapter 2, How to Think Critically.

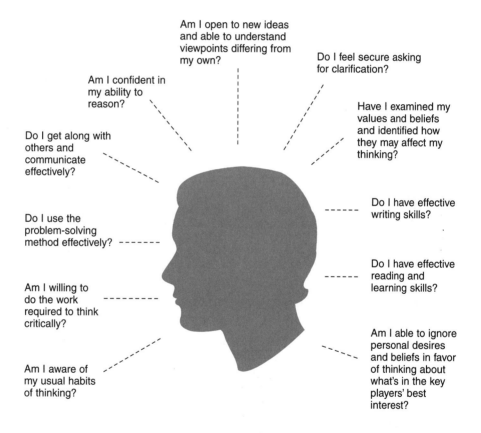

CRITICAL THINKING POTENTIAL

FIGURE 1–1

Questions to ask yourself to evaluate your potential to think critically.

OTHER PERSPECTIVES

Appreciation of Effort

"I'd rather have a basket of dandelions fresh-picked by a child, than the most beautiful bouquet of roses."   —*Susan Giedgowd, Mother, Teacher, and Leukemia Patient*

Critical Thinking Is More Than Problem Solving

Here's an example of critical thinking triggered by positive events. *When a baby is born in some hospitals, everyone shares in the celebration. With each birth the public address sys-*

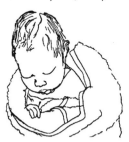

tem plays Brahms' Lullaby. Patients love it—even oncology patients, who say it lifts up their spirits and allows them to share someone else's joy. Parents who have just lost their baby are given the option of playing the lullaby or not. Many of them choose to have it played for their baby. "Playing the music is a simple thing that can be done for patients and families that costs virtually nothing and brings a great deal of pleasure."

—*Jean Young, ICU Patient Care Manager*

KEY POINTS

■ Critical thinking is purposeful and outcome directed (results oriented). To think critically in any situation, you must be clear about your *purpose:* What exactly are the results you want?

■ Because critical thinking is a complex activity that can be described in more than one way, there's no one *right* definition. Pages 8 and 9 provide some common descriptions of critical thinking and an applied definition for nursing.

■ Critical thinking is the key to resolving problems. Nurses who don't think critically become *part* of the problems.

■ Critical thinking is like any other skill (music, art, athletics). We each have our own styles and innate or learned capabilities. And we can all improve by gaining awareness, acquiring instruction, and consciously practicing to improve.

■ Considering the characteristics, or attitudes, of those who consistently demonstrate critical thinking gives you an overall picture of what it takes to think critically (see page 11).

■ In many ways, critical thinking is an upgraded version of problem solving. But besides problem solving, critical thinking focuses on gaining new knowledge and skills, seizing opportunities, and constantly finding ways to do things better.

■ Some people believe analytical thinking *is* critical thinking. However, critical thinking involves more than analyzing. It involves focusing on purpose, or desired results, and *drawing conclusions* about what you've analyzed.

■ There's a lot about critical thinking that you'll find similar to principles of science and the scientific method (see page 15).

■ We're only just beginning to learn how to maximize the human potential to think critically. Box 1–3 (page 16) gives an overview of what's new about critical thinking.

RECOMMENDATIONS FOR COMPLETING CRITICAL THINKING EXERCISES

1. Keep a record of your responses in a notebook or on a computer. Or if you want, tape record your responses. In some exercises, you may even choose to draw or diagram your response. Keeping all your responses together will give you a record you can review later to see how you've progressed. Since we'll go from simple to more complex ideas, you'll be surprised at the progress that will be evident when you review your responses later on.

2. At first, be more concerned with *substance* than grammar (as you would if you were writing a diary). However, as you progress, work to make your responses *clear to others*. Making your responses clear to others will help you clarify your thoughts.

3. If you have trouble *writing* and do better *verbally*, tape your response; then play it and write it down. This will save you time in the long run.

4. Don't be afraid to paraphrase: Paraphrasing helps you gain understanding because you explain what you read using familiar language (your own). To avoid concerns of plagiarism, cite the page numbers that you've chosen to paraphrase.

CRITICAL THINKING EXERCISES

1. Thinking critically about your reading requires you to personalize information or to make it your own by deciding how (or whether) it applies to you. Personalize the information in this chapter by answering the following questions:

   a. What information did you find to be most relevant or helpful?

   b. What information did you find least relevant or helpful?

   c. Think of at least two questions the information in this chapter raises for you.

2. Compare your responses to Exercise 1 with those of someone else who has read this chapter.

3. Complete the following sentences and then compare your responses with those of others:
   - *If I were to tell someone how I think, I would say that I . . .*

   - *I do my best thinking when . . .*

   - *I do my worst thinking when . . .*

4. Predict what could happen if someone who didn't think critically—someone who is self-focused—applied the rule below.*

   ▩ **Rule:** Critical thinking is purposeful and outcome directed (results oriented). To think critically in any situation, you must be clear about your *purpose:* What exactly are the results you want?

   ———————————

   *An example response for this exercise can be found in the Response Key at the back of the book beginning on page 238.

5. When you form an opinion, you draw a conclusion from facts or evidence.
   a. What's the difference between facts and opinions?*

   b. How can you determine if an opinion is valid?*

6. Think about the other perspective below. Discuss with a peer (or peers) the effect "mind games" (worrying too much or focusing on the negatives) can have on thinking and performance.

 OTHER PERSPECTIVES

You are your own coach . . .
"If you don't talk to yourself and give yourself pep talks, start now. Time was, only crazies talked to themselves; now, you miss the boat if you don't. Our minds are tricky things. We know now that attitude is the base on which knowledge and ability stand."   —*Jean T. Penny, PhD, ARNP, Consultant*

7. Consider Box 1–1 and Table 1–1 (page 5), addressing workplace skills. Identify three skills you'd like to improve; then think of some ways you can acquire the three skills you identified.

8. Complete the prechapter self-test, which has been reproduced below:
   a. Describe critical thinking using your own words, based on a commonly seen description of critical thinking.*
   b. Explain the difference between thinking and critical thinking.*
   c. Give at least three reasons why critical thinking is essential for nurses.*
   d. Explain the relationship between outcomes (results) and critical thinking.*
   e. Describe five critical thinking characteristics, traits, or dispositions you'd like to develop or improve.*
   f. Address how critical thinking is similar to and different from problem solving.*
   g. Identify four principles of the scientific method that are evident in critical thinking (see page 15).

---

*An example response for this exercise can be found in the Response Key at the back of the book beginning on page 238.

CRITICAL MOMENT

Being Creative and Applying Principles Works
Sometimes simple, principle-centered ideas get you the best results. Be creative and apply principles when searching for solutions.

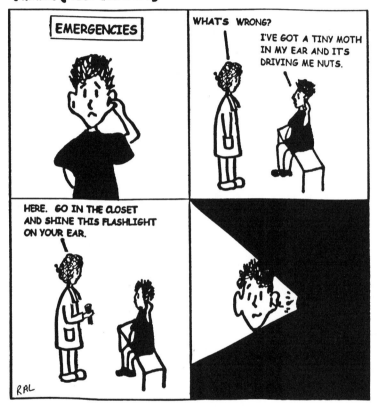

© R. Alfaro-LeFevre 1998.

Footnotes

[1]The Secretary's Commission on Achieving Necessary Skills [SCANS], The U.S. Department of Labor. (1992). *Learning a living: A blueprint for high performance, a SCANS report for America 2000* (p. xiv). Washington, D.C.: Author.

[2]Ennis, R., & Milman, J. (1985). *Cornell tests of critical thinking: Theory and practice* (pp. 9–26). Pacific Grove, CA: Midwest Publications.

[3]Paul, R. (1993). *Critical thinking: How to prepare students for a rapidly changing world.* Santa Rosa, CA: Foundation for Critical Thinking.

[4]Halpern, D. (1984). *Thought and knowledge.* Hillsdale, NJ: Lawrence Erlbaum Associates.

[5]Facione, N., Facione, P., & Sanchez, P. (1994). Critical thinking disposition as a measure of competent clinical judgment: The development of the California critical thinking disposition inventory. *Journal of Nursing Education, 33*(8), 345–350.

[6]American Psychological Association. (1990). Table I, Critical thinking: A statement of expert consensus for purposes of educational assessment and instruction. In *The APA Delphi Report.* Washington, D.C.: Author. (ERIC Document Reproduction Service No. 315 423).

[7]Colucciello, M. (1997). Critical thinking skills and dispositions of baccalaureate nursing students—A conceptual model for evaluation. *Journal of Professional Nursing, 13*(4), 236–245.

[8]Facione, P., & Facione, N. (1992). *The California critical thinking disposition inventory test manual.* Millbrae, CA: California Academia Press.

See comprehensive bibliography beginning on page 280.

2

How to Think Critically

Read the Learning Outcomes listed below and decide whether you can readily achieve each one. If you can, you don't need to read this chapter and can go on to Chapter 3. Don't be concerned if you can't achieve any of the outcomes at this time. We'll come back to these outcomes later in the chapter, in Critical Thinking Exercises.

LEARNING OUTCOMES

After completing this chapter, you should be able to:

- Give a description of how you think and learn and how it might be different from how other people think and learn.

- Explain how knowing personal styles can promote individual and group thinking.

- Discuss how human habits influence critical thinking ability.

- Explain the relationship between identifying outcomes and critical thinking.

- Give five strategies that enhance critical thinking and provide reasons why the strategies work.

- Explain why developing effective interpersonal and communication skills is essential to critical thinking.

- Identify the roles of logic, intuition, and trial and error in critical thinking.

- Describe at least five critical thinking skills you'd like to improve.

- Explain the relationship between critical thinking ability and developing character, knowledge, and skills.

ABSTRACT

Chapter 1 focused on *what* critical thinking is. This chapter focuses on *how* to think critically. It begins by pointing out the importance of connecting with personal thinking and learning styles. Then it examines factors influencing critical thinking, showing how being aware of these factors helps us improve. The importance of focusing on outcomes is stressed, and the roles of logic, intuition, and trial and error in critical thinking are discussed. General and specific critical thinking strategies are offered, including communication techniques that facilitate critical thinking. Finally, it addresses the need to master specific intellectual skills and points out the importance of maintaining high standards and developing a critical thinking character.

GAINING INSIGHT

In Chapter 1 you had the opportunity to focus on the first step to learning how to think critically: gaining insight into *what* critical thinking is. This chapter takes you on to the next step: developing awareness of *how* to think critically. As you read this chapter, keep the following in mind:

- Thinking is a skill like any other (music, art, athletics).
- As with any skill, we each have our own styles and innate or learned capabilities.
- We can all improve by gaining insight, acquiring instruction and feedback, and consciously practicing to improve.

WHAT'S YOUR PERSONAL STYLE AND WHY DOES IT MATTER?

Developing an awareness of your personal style—how and why you think and learn the way you do—is an excellent starting point for improving thinking. Research on thinking and learning styles is growing. We now know that many people who consider themselves to be poor thinkers or learners are not so at all. They simply haven't learned to use their own natural abilities.

Most experts agree there are two important factors that determine whether you think and learn well. You must:

1. Believe in your ability to be a good thinker and learner.
2. Be willing to master strategies that can help you think and learn more efficiently *in your own way.*

Understanding Learning Style Differences

If you're one of the millions of people who believe that they aren't good learners, it may be that you haven't had the opportunity to learn in the ways that are best for you. Remember the following:

▨ **Rule: There are no learning disabilities or right or wrong ways to learn—there are only differences.** Each of us is responsible for connecting with our preferred styles and mastering strategies that can help us learn efficiently in our *own* way.

If you aren't keenly aware of how you learn best—for example, whether you're a doer, observer, listener, or whatever—review pages 253 and 254, which give an overview of various learning styles. Critical thinking focuses on achieving desired outcomes efficiently. You're using critical thinking when you identify ways you can think and learn more efficiently.

Connecting with Personality Types

Each of us is born with a specific personality that plays a major role in how we think. Your personality determines what information you notice and recall, the way you make decisions, and even how much structure and control you prefer. Connecting with your own particular personality type helps you gain insight into how and why you think the way you do. It helps you get in touch with your talents and blind spots and find ways to improve. Understanding personality types different from your own helps you realize how and why *others* think the way *they* do. Armed with this information, you can facilitate "meetings of the minds."

Boxes 2–1 and 2–2 give summaries of two different and complementary ways of describing personality. Box 2–1 addresses the *Myers-Briggs Type Indicator,* which helps you examine your style based on the work of psychologist Carl Jung. Box 2–2 addresses the *Hartman Personality Profile,* a simple but powerful tool that helps you connect with what *motivates* you in life. As you look at these style descriptions, keep in mind that no one style is better than another. They are all good styles, each having specific strengths and limitations. What's important is that you know that there are distinct style differences and that you connect with

BOX 2–1	**What's Your Thinking Style?* Myers-Briggs Type Indicator**

Extrovert

- Thinks out loud
- Draws energy from being with people

Sensate

- Perceives the word discretely through the five senses
- Looks for facts

Thinking

- Uses objective data
- Seeks just decisions

Judging

- Orders the environment
- Likes to plan

Introvert

- Thinks inside
- Draws energy from being quiet

Intuitive

- Perceives the world overall
- Looks for meaning

Feeling

- Uses subjective data
- Seeks fair decisions

Perceiving

- Keeps things flexible and open
- Likes to be spontaneous

*See page 255 for recommended reading for personal application of personality type.

From Schoessler, M., Conedera, F., Bell, L., et al. (1993). Use of the Myers-Briggs type indicator to develop a continuing education department. *Journal of Nursing Staff Development, 9*(1), 9.

your own style, celebrating the strengths and developing strategies to overcome limitations.*

OTHER PERSPECTIVES

Nobody's Perfect

"I thought everyone talked to themselves with a tremendous amount of harshness and called themselves 'losers' and 'stupid.' I had to learn to allow myself to make a mistake without becoming defensive and unforgiving."

—Lisa Kudrow, Actor

---

*The summaries of personality types provided in this book are intended to give you a *beginning awareness* of personality types. To fully understand how to apply principles of personality type, you *must* do more in-depth study. For example, read the suggested readings accompanying each summary, hire an expert, or attend a training session.

BOX 2–2   **What Motivates You? Hartman Personality Profile**

According to Taylor Hartman, psychologist, leadership coach, and author of *The Color Code,* how we think and interact with others is greatly affected by our innate personality: we're each born with a specific motive or inner drive—an intense need to operate from a certain perspective. For example, consider the motives of the four personality types represented by each of his "colors" below:

Reds

These people are born with the drive for **power and productivity.** Some of their strengths are that they're logical, confident, determined, visionary individuals who take charge and make things happen. Some of their limitations are that they tend to be arrogant, bossy, impatient, argumentative, and very focused on themselves.

Blues

These people are born with the drive for **intimacy and closeness.** They want to get to really *know* people, have very strong *feelings,* and enjoy talking about daily details of life. Some of their strengths are that they are creative, caring, understanding people who are reliable, loyal, and sincere. Some of their limitations are that they tend to be judgmental, worry prone, doubtful, and moody and to have unrealistic expectations.

Whites

These people are born with the drive for **peace and harmony.** Some of their strengths are that they're kind, tolerant, easy-going people who are patient, insightful, and diplomatic. Some of their limitations are that they tend to avoid conflict at all costs and are indecisive and silently stubborn. They may also explode (usually because their need for peace causes them to hold things inside until there are so many things bothering them that one more problem is too much for them to take).

Yellows

These people are born with the drive to **have fun and enjoy life in the present moment.** Some of their strengths are that they're outgoing, enthusiastic, optimistic, popular, and trusting. They are simply fun to be around. Some of their limitations are that they tend to avoid facing facts and can be impulsive, undisciplined, disorganized, and uncommitted.

Want to Know More?

The Color Code provides a 45-question profile you can take to find out which of the four different color-coded personality types—Red, Blue, White, or Yellow—is your *true* color. It helps you connect with natural strengths and limitations and teaches you how to maximize potential. Also recommended: *The Character Code.* Appendix C, page 255, provides recommended readings for personal application of personality types.

Summarized from Hartman, T. (1998). *The color code.* New York: Scribner.

FACTORS INFLUENCING CRITICAL THINKING ABILITY

Have you ever found yourself saying, "I just wasn't thinking right" or, better, "Boy, that really got me thinking—I came up with some great ideas"? We've all felt this way at one time or another. Our ability to think well varies, depending on personal factors and circumstances that are evident at the time. For example, look at Table 2–1, which lists factors usu-

TABLE 2–1	**Factors Influencing Critical Thinking Ability**
FACTORS **USUALLY ENHANCING** CRITICAL THINKING	FACTORS **USUALLY IMPEDING** CRITICAL THINKING
Personal Factors	*Personal Factors*
Moral development (fair-mindedness)	Dislikes, prejudices, biases
Age (older you are)	Lack of self-confidence
Self-confidence*	Limited knowledge of problem solving, decision making, and research principles
Emotional intelligence	
Knowledge of problem solving, decision making, and research principles	Poor communication skills
	Limited early evaluation
Effective communication and interpersonal skills	Poor writing skills
	Poor reading and learning skills
Habitual early evaluation	
Past experience*	*Situational Factors*
Effective writing skills	Anxiety, stress, or fatigue
Effective reading and learning skills	Evaluative or judgmental styles
	Lack of motivation
Situational Factors	Limited knowledge of related factors
Knowledge of related factors	Lack of awareness of resources
Awareness of resources	Time limitations†
Awareness of risks*	Environmental distractions
Positive reinforcement	
Presence of motivating factors	

*Sometimes may *impede* critical thinking (see text on pages 31 to 36).
†Sometimes may *enhance* critical thinking (see text on page 36).

ally enhancing critical thinking and those usually impeding critical thinking. Then read on for an explanation of *how and why* these factors are so influential.

Personal Factors

Moral Development (Fair-mindedness). Many experts cite a positive correlation between moral development and critical thinking ability: People with a mature level of moral development—those with a clear, carefully reasoned sense of *what's right, wrong, and fair*—are more likely to think critically. It makes sense that those who are keenly aware of their values and beliefs and consistently approach situations with an attitude of "I must consider all viewpoints and make decisions *in the key players' best interest,*" already are critical thinkers.

Age. Most authors agree that age also correlates with critical thinking ability: the older you get, the better thinker you become. There are two logical reasons for this:

1. Moral development usually comes with maturity.
2. Most older people have had more opportunities to practice reasoning in different situations.

Dislikes, Prejudices, and Biases. These can be subtle but powerful factors that *hinder* critical thinking. If you're unable to recognize and overcome these factors, it will be difficult to think critically in situations where you have to function in spite of your dislikes, prejudices, and biases.

Emotional Intelligence. This is the ability to make emotions work in positive ways, and it enhances critical thinking. *How* you feel about something has tremendous influence over *what* you think. However, all too often, you aren't even aware of deep, strong feelings. Connecting with emotions and giving them the attention they deserve—making them explicit, accepting them, and recognizing their influence over thinking—helps us adjust and get better results. Box 2–3 (page 32) gives strategies for using emotional intelligence to promote critical thinking.

Self-confidence. For the most part, self-confidence aids critical thinking. If you aren't confident, you use much of your brainpower worrying about failure, reducing the energy available for *productive thinking.* Occasionally self-confidence is an *impeding* factor: Some become so *overly con-*

BOX 2–3	**Using Emotional Intelligence to Promote Critical Thinking**

1. **Connect with emotions.** Put your feelings into words and, through dialogue, help others to do the same ("I feel . . . because . . ."). Never assume you know what someone else is feeling or expect others to know what you're feeling.
2. **Accept true feelings for what they are.** No one's to blame for what he or she feels.
3. **Master mood management.** Recognize the importance of connecting with how emotions are affecting thinking. Learn how to manage feelings like anger, anxiety, fear, and discouragement.
4. **Don't be too concerned with isolated events.** Patterns of behavior are what matter. (Don't sweat the small stuff.)
5. **Keep in mind that emotions are "catching."** If you're depressed, you may trigger depression in someone else. If you're enthusiastic, you may trigger enthusiasm.
6. **Do something to reduce stress.** Take time out, use humor, play a game, take a walk, learn to use yoga or guided imagery.

Recommended reading: Weisinger, H. (1998). *Emotional intelligence at work.* San Francisco, CA: Jossey-Bass.

fident that they believe they can't be wrong or that they have little to learn from others.

Knowledge of Problem Solving, Decision Making, Nursing Process, and Research Principles. Because critical thinking is based on many of these same principles, familiarity with the methods *enhances* critical thinking.

Effective Communication and Interpersonal Skills. Developing effective communication and interpersonal skills is essential to critical thinking. You must be able to understand others, be understood by others, and gain others' trust to get the facts required for sound reasoning. Keep in mind that communication is more than talking and listening: You need to consider the messages you send by your *behavior* over a period of time. Box 2–4, pages 33–34, gives communication strategies enhancing critical thinking.

Habitual Early Evaluation. When you evaluate early, checking whether your information is accurate, complete, and up-to-date, you're able to make corrections *early*. You avoid making risky decisions based on outdated, inaccurate, or incomplete information. When you evaluate early by comparing your progress with a written plan, you're better able to stay

| BOX 2–4 | **Communication Strategies Enhancing Critical Thinking** |

- Seek First to Understand, Then to be Understood™ (Covey, 1989).
- Clearly state that your intent is not to *judge* but to *understand* (e.g., "I'm not here to judge. I just want to understand what's going on").
- Use strategies that help you see other points of view.
  - Ask for clarification. For example, "I don't mean to be difficult, but I still don't understand. Can you clarify further?"
  - Use phrases like, from your way of looking at it . . . or from your perspective. For example, "*From your perspective,* how do you see this situation?"
  - Paraphrase in your own words. For example, "It seems to me that you're saying. . . . Is that correct?"
- Listen empathetically (with the intent of understanding the other person's way of looking at the world). This is often called trying to imagine what it would be like to "walk in someone else's shoes." Listening empathetically requires four steps:
  1. Clear your mind of thoughts about how you view the situation or concerns about how you're going to respond.
  2. Focus on listening to the person's feelings and perceptions.
  3. Rephrase the feelings and perceptions as you understand them to be.
  4. Detach and come back to your own frame of reference.
- Apply strategies that help you get accurate and comprehensive information.
  - Use open-ended questions (those requiring more than a one-word answer). For example, How do you feel about leaving tomorrow?
  - Avoid closed-ended question (those requiring only a one-word answer). For example, Are you ready to leave tomorrow?
  - Use exploratory statements that lead the person to expand on certain issues. For example, Tell me more about. . . .
  - Don't use leading questions (those that lead someone to a desired answer). For example, You don't smoke, do you?
  - Put body language into words. For example, You looked a little sad. . . .
  - Use silence. Allow the person time to gather his thoughts.
  - Remember the value of using written communication (letters and diaries really help).
    · Record the information you gathered; then look to see what's missing and check for inconsistencies.
    · Ask the person to keep a log or diary or keep one yourself.

Box continued on following page

BOX 2–4	**Communication Strategies Enhancing Critical Thinking** *Continued*

- Use strategies that help you get your point across.
  - Make sure the time and place are appropriate.
  - Wait until the person is ready to listen.
  - When voicing an opinion, use phrases that convey that you're *voicing an opinion*, rather than dictating what is so (e.g., From my way of looking at it. . . . From my perspective. . . .)
  - Ask the person to paraphrase what you've said (e.g., I need to know you understand. Explain to me what I just said.).
- Be cognizant of others' communication styles rather than trying to force them to use yours (e.g., don't use touch, even if you like to, if the other person seems to recoil from touch; if someone is formal and reserved, respect his style).
- Exhibit behaviors that send messages like, I'm responsible, I can be trusted, and I want to do a good job. For example, keep promises, be punctual, accept responsibility, and respect others' time.
- Acknowledge and apologize when you've caused inconvenience, been careless or made a mistake, or offended someone.
- Respect others' territory; ask permission (e.g., May I listen to your chest? rather than, Sit up and let me listen to your chest).

See also Communicating Bad News, pages 192 to 194.

on your intended path—your brain often doesn't notice when you've "gone off on a tangent." For example, if I hadn't consistently checked to be sure that I followed the plan I developed for this book, I can assure you, you'd be reading some lengthy discussions that would be interesting to *me* but irrelevant and boring for *you!*

Past Experience. Most authors view this as an enhancing factor: Experienced nurses usually are more able to think critically because they have previous job-specific problem-solving knowledge. Sometimes, however, past experience is an *impeding* factor: You become a victim of tunnel vision, seeing only what you expect to see. If your past experience is *different* from the present situation, you may have trouble thinking critically. A classic example of this is when a psychiatric nurse fails to consider whether someone's confusion could be related to a *medical problem*, and vice versa (a medical-surgical nurse fails to consider whether someone's confusion could be related to a *psychiatric problem*).

Effective Writing Skills. These promote critical thinking. When you learn how to make yourself clear in writing, you learn to apply critical thinking principles like identifying an organized approach, deciding what's relevant, and focusing on others' perspectives.

Effective Reading and Learning Skills. These are enhancing factors. Because critical thinking often requires that you use resources independently, you must know how to read and learn well. Having effective reading skills doesn't mean knowing how to read *rapidly*. It means taking the time to identify what's important, drawing conclusions about what the material implies, and considering how it applies to the real world.

Situational Factors

Anxiety, Stress, Fatigue. For the most part, these *reduce* your thinking power. High levels of anxiety and stress, often the first to tap your brain energy, make concentration difficult. When you're fatigued, you're already operating on a "low battery." A *low* anxiety level, however, like being a little nervous about a test, can *promote* critical thinking by motivating you to prepare.

Awareness of Risks Involved. Usually this is an *enhancing* factor. When you know the risks, you think more carefully, making sure you've made a prudent decision before acting. Sometimes awareness of the risks can increase anxiety to a level that *impedes* critical thinking. For example, remember how hard it was to think well when you gave your first injection.

Knowledge of Related Factors. The more you know about a situation, the better you'll be able to reason. For example, you might know about diabetes, but if you don't know the *person* you're going to teach—know the person's lifestyle, desires, and motivations—you'll be unlikely to design a plan of care that the person will follow.

Awareness of Resources. Awareness of *resources* allows us to think critically, even with limited knowledge. For example, nurses frequently think critically about drug administration with limited drug-specific knowledge. They check with resources like pharmacists and drug manuals before giving unfamiliar drugs (e.g., they find out usual dose range, contraindications, and possible side effects).

Positive Reinforcement. This *promotes* critical thinking by helping you build self-confidence and focus on what you're doing *right*.

Evaluative or Judgmental Styles. Those who convey an evaluative or judgmental style usually *impede* critical thinking. People who feel they're being evaluated or judged often spend more energy worrying about what *others* are thinking than what *they're* thinking.

Presence of Motivating Factors. Factors that motivate you to *want* to think critically aid thinking because they connect with your desires, enticing you to get your brain "in gear." It's important to remember that what motivates you might not motivate *someone else*. An example of a *common* motivating factor for critical thinking is knowing *why* you're asked to do or study something (knowing why the action is important or knowing how it's useful).

Time Limitations. This can be an *enhancing or impeding* factor. Time limitations, when realistic, are motivating factors: Deadlines stimulate us to get going and get things done. If there's *too little time*, however, you may make decisions quicker than you'd like and come up with less than satisfactory answers. It's interesting to note that the courts recognize that time limitations influence our thinking. Courts give more leeway to decisions that were made in emergency situations than to those made with plenty of time for thinking.

Environmental Distractions. These impede critical thinking for obvious reasons—the more distractions there are, the more difficult it is to stay focused.

Habits Causing Barriers to Critical Thinking

Okay. We've now covered factors influencing critical thinking ability. However, I've saved a major factor for a separate discussion: The *human factor*.

As *humans*, we have many wonderful qualities—qualities that separate us from other life on this planet. As humans, however, we also instinctually develop habits that help us feel better about ourselves—habits that protect us for the moment but hinder our potential to think critically *in the long run.* Let's take a look at some common human habits that create barriers to critical thinking.

Vincent Ruggiero says there are six habits that hinder thinking: *mine-is-better, face-saving, resistance to change, conformity, stereotyping,* and *self-deception.** I like to add another one: *the choosing-only-one habit.* Following is a discussion of each of these habits. Consider each one in relation to yourself and others you know. Keep in mind that we're all human and that most of these habits are simply a result of human nature. Whether we realize it or not, we're all victims of these behaviors to some extent at one time or another.

Mine-Is-Better. We all tend to regard our ideas, values, religions, cultures, and points of view as being superior to others. To enhance your potential for critical thinking, you need to consciously work to control this habit as you search for truth.

Choosing-Only-One. When faced with two choices, we tend to choose *only one* of the two. We forget to think about things like, Are there other, better choices? Can we do both? Can we do neither? Beginners are usually the most vulnerable to the choosing-only-one habit. They tend to blindly accept that if they've chosen one of two choices, then they've made a good decision. They also tend to make the common assumption that there must be one best way to do this, rather than, there probably are several good ways of doing this, and each has its advantages and disadvantages. We can overcome this tendency by remembering to ask ourselves, Must I choose only one? or Is this the only way?

Face-saving. When we find that we've done or said something wrong, we have a strong instinct to protect our image—we try to save face. Critical thinking requires that we learn and grow. As we learn and grow, we'll make mistakes or realize our old ways of thinking or doing things can be improved. To be a critical thinker, we must learn to be comfortable saying things like, I'm not sure, I was wrong, or I have to think about that.

---

*Ruggiero, V. (1991). *The Art of Thinking: A Guide to Critical and Creative Thought* (3rd ed.). Glenview, IL: HarperCollins.

Resistance to Change. While most of us realize change usually occurs for good reasons, we tend to resist it. All too often change is considered "guilty until proven innocent." We reject new ideas and ways without examining them fairly. Overcoming this barrier doesn't mean embracing every new idea uncritically. It means being willing to suspend judgment long enough to make an informed decision on whether the change is worthwhile.

Conformity. While some conformity, like following policies and procedures, is good, we sometimes engage in *harmful conformity.* Harmful conformity is when we conform to group thinking rather than *think independently* to avoid being viewed as being "different." Conforming without thought stifles the ability to be creative and improve. An example of conformity that *may* be harmful is supporting a political leader simply because of peer pressure rather than seeking to understand the policies supported by the leader.

Stereotyping. We stereotype when we make fixed and unbending overgeneralizations about others (e.g., homeless people aren't very bright). When our minds are fixed and unbending, we may not see what's really before us. By recognizing our tendency to stereotype, we can make a conscious effort to overcome this habit, which distorts our view of reality.

Self-deception. This is the purposeful forgetting of things about ourselves we don't particularly feel good about. An example of this is experienced nurses who deceive themselves into believing they were never as shy, nervous, or insecure as the students they encounter today.

Summary

To summarize, being aware of habits and factors influencing critical thinking helps us identify strategies that promote critical thinking. For example, if we know anxiety and stress impede critical thinking, we know we need to *reduce anxiety and stress* to enhance critical thinking. As humans, we might all be victims of deeply ingrained habits of mine-is-better, choosing-only-one, resistance to change, face-saving, conformity, stereotyping, and self-deception. It's simply human nature. As humans, however, we can overcome these barriers by becoming aware of our human ways and working to replace old patterns with new ways of responding.

Covey's 7 Habits of Highly Effective People

Steven Covey, author of the highly successful book *The 7 Habits of Highly Effective People*, also addresses the importance of replacing old patterns with new habits. He offers seven habits that can help us be more productive as individuals and more successful in creating positive interpersonal relationships. These habits, listed below, enhance critical thinking because critical thinking depends on our ability to nurture the interpersonal relationships required to gain information and work as a team.*

1. **Be Proactive®**. Choose to be responsible for your own life, anticipate responses, and act before things happen.
2. **Begin With the End in Mind®**. Develop goals and make your expectations explicit.
3. **Put First Things First®**. Decide what's important and stick to priorities moment by moment, day by day.
4. **Think Win-Win®**. Seek *mutual benefit* in all human interactions.
5. **Seek First to Understand, Then to be Understood®**. Communicate effectively.
6. **Synergize®**. Recognize that the whole is greater than the sum of its parts: collaborate, bringing diverse ideas and talents together to create new and better ideas.
7. **Sharpen the Saw®**. Look after yourself physically, emotionally, and spiritually. (Covey explains *Sharpening the Saw* by telling a story about a man who is sawing a tree trunk for hours: The saw is dull, and the man is exhausted. Someone suggests that he might do better if he sharpens the saw. The man responds, "I don't have time" and continues to work ineffectively.)

---

*Summarized from Covey, S. (1989). *The 7 Habits of Highly Effective People.* New York: Simon & Schuster, © 1989 Stephen R. Covey. Used with permission of Franklin Covey Co. All trademarks of Franklin Covey are used with permission. All rights reserved. www.FranklinCovey.com

CRITICAL THINKING EXERCISES

1. Study Boxes 2–1 (What's Your Thinking Style?) and 2–2 (What Motivates You?).* In a group or in a personal journal, discuss:
   a. Your thoughts about your thinking style and main motive according to Myers-Briggs and Hartman.
   b. How your style and motive affect your ability to think clearly.
   c. How working with people with styles different than your own affects your thinking.
   d. How you would feel about taking one of the personality tests for your own personal knowledge versus for use at school or work.
2. How does knowing your preferred learning style influence your ability to think critically?†

3. What would you say is your preferred learning style? (If you don't know, study pages 253 and 254.)

4. a. Emotive thinking is thinking that's driven by feelings. How does this relate to critical thinking?†

   b. Write a paragraph explaining how intelligent use of emotions can facilitate better thinking.†

   c. In a personal journal, write about the influence of feelings on your thinking (for example, whether you are ruled more by your heart than your head, or vice versa, and what difference that makes). Identify at least one thing you can do to improve your

---

*Also recommended: Schoessler, M., Conedera, F., Bell, L., et al. (1993). Use of the Meyer-Briggs type indicator to develop a continuing education department. *Journal of Nursing Staff Development, 9*(1), 8–13.

†An example response for this exercise can be found in the Response Key at the back of the book beginning on page 238.

ability to have more balanced thinking (thinking that considers both "heart" and "head").

5. Respond to the following from the prechapter self-test:
   a. Give a description of how you think and learn and how it might be different from how other people think and learn.
   b. Explain how knowing personal styles promotes individual and group thinking.*
   c. Discuss how human habits influence critical thinking ability.*

Now that we've addressed factors influencing critical thinking, (personal and situational factors, habits, and personality types), let's go on to consider how identifying clear outcomes improves ability to think critically.

---

*An example response for this exercise can be found in the Response Key at the back of the book beginning on page 238.

GOALS VERSUS OUTCOMES

The words *goal* and *outcome* are often used interchangeably. Although these two terms do have similar meanings, there is a significant difference. Remember the following rule:

▓ **Rules**
- Use **goal** when stating **general intent** (what you aim to do). *Example:* My goal is to improve my Spanish by next year.
- Use **outcome** to describe **specific results** that will be observed at a certain point in time when the goal is achieved. *Example:* By next September, I'll be able to speak Spanish well enough to demonstrate fluency when interviewing for bilingual nursing positions.

Understanding the above relationship between goals and outcomes helps you think more critically. Goal statements, because they focus on *intent,* may be vague, lofty, and unrealistic. Have you ever had great intentions, done a lot of work, and then found out too late that you didn't really think things through? Outcome statements, because they center on *clearly observable results,* force you to think things through, helping you be realistic and focused from the start.

Outcome-focused (Results-oriented) Thinking

To promote outcome-focused (results-oriented) thinking, there are certain principles you need to apply. Outcomes should be:

- **Well reasoned** (e.g., they should be realistic, considering the key players capabilities and available time and resources)
- **Clearly stated** in terms that describe the results that will be observed when the outcomes are reached (they should answer the questions, who, what, how much, how well, under what circumstances, and by when).

Are you thinking the above is pretty obvious? Perhaps so, but it's not as simple as that. All too often we *think* we've clearly identified what we want to accomplish, but we're vague about exactly how we'll measure success. We have a human tendency to focus more on what we're *aiming to do* than on what's actually being *accomplished*.

Determining outcomes is a skill that requires practice. Pages 173 to 176 (Chapter 5) address how to develop specific client-centered outcomes and provide opportunities to practice writing outcomes. For now, just remember that if you haven't given enough thought to exactly what outcome you expect to achieve and how you'll evaluate whether the outcome is achieved, you aren't thinking critically.

Below are examples of questions you need to ask and answer to stay focused on outcomes.

Question	Example Answer
What exactly is my desired outcome (result or purpose)?	The paper I write will meet course requirements and get an A.
How will I determine the likelihood of achieving my desired outcome (getting an A)?	I'll compare final draft with the assignment requirements and decide whether I've paid attention to the most important requirements.
Exactly what will be able to be observed when I achieve my desired outcome?	The grade I receive on the paper will be an A.

CRITICAL MOMENT

Imagine the Consequences

Once I was on a planning committee for a conference. One of our goals was to keep costs down, so we decided to skip refreshments for the afternoon break. This seemed to make sense until someone put her mind in the future and said, "Well, I don't want to be the one who has to stand up in front of 500 tired, thirsty people and announce, 'there will be no refreshments during this break.'" After that comment, we changed our minds. When determining outcomes, "think future." Imagine consequences: exactly how things will be on the day you reach your outcome.

CRITICAL THINKING STRATEGIES

This section first considers general strategies promoting critical thinking, then goes on to look at specific strategies.

Nine Key Questions

Have you ever heard the saying, It's not what you know but what you know to *ask* that matters? Nine key questions can help you determine your approach to critical thinking in different situations. These are summarized in Box 2–5 and addressed in more depth on page 44.

1. **What major outcomes (results) do I/we hope to achieve?** You'll think more critically if you can clearly describe what everyone can expect to observe when you achieve your goal.

BOX 2–5	**Nine Key Critical Thinking Questions**

1. What **major outcomes** (results) do I/we hope to achieve?
2. What **problems or issues** must be addressed to achieve the major outcomes?
3. What are the **circumstances** (what is the context)?
4. What **knowledge** is required?
5. How much room is there for **error**?
6. How much **time** do I/we have?
7. What **resources** can help?
8. Whose **perspectives** must be considered?
9. What's **influencing thinking**?

■ **Memory jog.** Use the following sentence to remember the above questions (the first letter of each word below corresponds with the above bold-type words): **M**ost **p**eople **c**an **k**now **e**very **t**ime **r**esources **p**rovide **i**nformation.

2. **What problems or issues must be addressed to achieve the major outcomes?** You need to prevent, control, or resolve these to achieve the outcomes.

3. **What are the circumstances (what is the context)?** The approach to critical thinking varies, depending on the circumstances (context). For example, you're in a classroom and the instructor asks you how you would manage a patient in shock. You aren't sure, but you *think* you know, so it's appropriate for you to answer. If you're in the clinical area, however, trying to manage this problem alone based on uncertain knowledge is inappropriate.

4. **What knowledge is required?** Discipline-specific theoretical and experiential knowledge is essential to being able to think critically. For example, how can you think critically about managing cardiac pain if you don't know the causes and common treatments of cardiac pain? If you don't know what knowledge is required, you probably don't know enough to achieve your goal—you must get help.

5. **How much room is there for error?** When there's less room for error, we must carefully assess the situation, examine *all possible solutions*, and make every effort to make prudent decisions. For example, which situation below has less room for error, and how might your approach to decision making differ in each situation?

   a. You're trying to decide whether to give an over-the-counter antihistamine to someone who's been in excellent health but who's been having trouble sleeping.

   b. You're trying to decide whether to give an over-the-counter antihistamine to someone with multiple health problems.

   Obviously, situation *a* has more room for error because the person is healthy and therefore less likely to have preexisting conditions that might be aggravated by the antihistamine. In situation *b*, unlike situation *a*, you need to consult the person's attending physician.

6. **How much time do I/we have?** If we have plenty of time to make a decision, we can take time to think independently, using resources such as textbooks to guide our thinking. If we don't have much time, we may be required to refer the problem to an expert immediately to expedite care delivery.

7. **What resources can help?** Identifying resources (textbooks, computers, expert clinicians) is essential to accessing the information you need to think critically. For example, most nurses don't know every hospital policy by heart. Rather, they know what situations are covered by policies and refer to the policy manual as needed.

8. **Whose perspectives must be considered?** Efficient solutions must consider the perspectives of all of the key players involved or you risk having conflicting purposes. For example, to develop an effective plan for home care, you must consider the perspectives of the patient, other household members, and other key members of the health care team. Imagine what could happen if you sent a grandmother home with lots of brightly colored medications and everyone forgot to consider the perspective of a toddler in the home!

9. **What's influencing thinking?** Recognizing influencing factors (for example, personal beliefs and biases) helps us be objective and find ways to compensate for factors that might impede our ability to think clearly. For example, a nurse who is strongly against abortion would be wise to avoid working in gynecology, where women's decisions might make it difficult to give nursing care objectively.

Using Logic, Intuition, and Trial and Error

Let's consider when and how to use logic, intuition, and trial and error.

Logic, or sound reasoning that's based on evidence, is the foundation for critical thinking. It's the safest and most reliable strategy for problem solving and therefore should be used when making all important decisions.

Intuition is best described as knowing something without evidence. The most effective use of intuition is to use it *as a guide to look for evidence.* For example, if your intuition tells you something is wrong with someone, regard this feeling as a "red flag" that says "Watch this person closely" or "Get an expert here quickly to check this person." Using intuition is a valuable strategy for problem solving, especially for experienced nurses, who may subconsciously recall a wide range of experiences. Before you *act* on intuition alone, however—before you act on gut feelings that aren't supported by evidence—be sure your actions won't cause harm.

Trial and error, or trying several solutions until one that works is found, is a *risky* but sometimes necessary approach to problem solving. Trial and error should be used *only* when there's plenty of room for error, when the problem can be monitored closely, and when the solutions have been logically thought through. An example of when trial and error is commonly used in nursing is in trying to determine the best way for a sterile dressing to be applied to an active person's wound: Often it takes several tries before the best way can be determined.

Focusing on the Big and Small Picture

There's a trend to emphasize the importance of focusing on the "big picture" (the whole) rather than the "small picture" (the parts, the details). Usually we need to do *both,* however, if we want to think critically. Consider the following examples.

- Mr. Juarez is in the coronary care unit and tells you he's experiencing chest pain. Treating both "the whole" (Mr. Juarez's pain and anxiety) and "the parts" (Mr. Juarez's oxygen-deprived heart) is essential to resolving the chest pain (and, perhaps, to saving his life).
- You're trying to teach Tonya how to care for her newborn. You're well prepared with lots of nice pamphlets. She seems interested, but she keeps yawning and doesn't seem to retain information very long. Finally you say, "Is there a better time we could do this?" She admits that she hasn't slept all night and is extremely fatigued. You come back later after Tonya's had a good rest. She learns readily. In this case, paying attention to an important *detail* (the fact that she was tired) helped you be a more effective teacher.

Remember to ask questions like, What's the big picture here? Am I considering both the parts and the whole? and Am I paying attention to key details?

Specific Strategies

Several authors have cited simple, specific strategies to facilitate critical thinking in any situation. These are summarized below.

- **Anticipate the questions others might ask** (for example, What will my instructor want to know? or What will the doctor want to know?). This helps identify a wider scope of questions that need to be answered to gain relevant information.
- **Ask what-else questions.** For example, change Have we done everything? to What else do we need to do? Asking what-else questions pushes you to look further and be more complete.
- **Think out loud or write your thoughts down.** When you put your thinking into words, you make your ideas, reasons, and logic explicit, making it easier to evaluate and correct yourself.
- **Ask an expert to think out loud.** When you ask experts to think out loud, you often learn organized systematic approaches to solving problems and making decisions.

- **Ask what-if questions** like, What if the worst happens? or What if we try another way? This helps you be proactive instead of reactive. It enhances your creativity and helps you put things in perspective.
- **Ask why** (determine underlying reasons). To fully understand something, you must know *what* it is and *why* it's so. There's a saying, "She who knows what and how is likely to get a good job. She who knows *why* is likely to be her boss."
- **Paraphrase in your own words.** Paraphrasing helps you understand information using a familiar language (your own).
- **Compare and contrast.** This forces you to look closely at the *parts* of something as well as the *whole,* helping you get more familiar with both things you're comparing. For example, if I asked you to compare two different kinds of apples, you'd have to *look closely at both of them.* As a result of comparing them, you'd also be more likely to know and *remember* each type of apple better.
- **Organize and reorganize information.** Organizing information helps you see certain patterns, but it may make you *miss* others. Reorganizing information helps you see some of those *other* patterns. For example, compare the group of numbers in *a* below with the group of numbers listed in *b* and *c* below (each group contains the same numbers, organized differently). What patterns do you see and which is easier to remember?
  a. 36345643   b. 34343 656   c. 333 44 566
- **Look for flaws in your thinking.** Ask questions like, What's missing? and How could this be made better? If you don't go looking for flaws, you'll be unlikely to find them. Once you've found them, you can make corrections early.
- **Ask someone else to look for flaws in your thinking.** This offers a "fresh eye" for evaluation and may bring new ideas and perspectives.
- **Develop good habits of inquiry** (habits that aid in the search for the truth, such as keeping an open mind, verifying information, and taking enough time).
- **Revisit information.** When you come back and look at something after a period of time, you'll be likely to view it differently.
- **Replace the phrases I don't know or I'm not sure with I need to find out.** This demonstrates you have the confidence and ability to find answers and mobilizes you to locate resources.
- **Turn errors into learning opportunities.** We all make mistakes. They're stepping stones to maturity and new ideas. If you aren't making any mistakes, maybe you aren't trying enough new things.

- **Share your mistakes—they're** VALUABLE. Sharing your mistakes helps others avoid making the same mistake and may identify common misconceptions or problems that need to be rectified.

CRITICAL THINKING SKILLS

Experts have identified certain skills that must be mastered to think critically. Although it's beyond the scope of this discussion to address *all* of these skills, below is a list of skills commonly used in nursing. Read through this list, asking yourself two questions as you consider each one:

1. How often do I use this skill in everyday situations?
2. Would I know how to do this in a specific nursing situation?

- **Identifying assumptions:** Recognizing when something is presented as fact, without proof. *Example:* Someone reports to you that a surgical patient is having incisional pain. You ask, "What is the pain like?" and the person responds, "I didn't ask, but he had surgery this morning, so it's got to be his incision." In fact, the pain could be related to any number of problems, ranging from a severe headache to a heart attack.
- **Identifying an organized approach to assessment:** Choosing a systematic approach that enhances ability to collect all the relevant data. *Example:* Performing a physical examination using a head-to-toe approach (carefully examining the head, then the neck, then the trunk and arms, and so on, down to the toes).
- **Checking accuracy and reliability:** Verifying information to be sure it's factual. *Example:* Double-checking an infant's weight when it's significantly different from the previous weight measurements.
- **Distinguishing relevant from irrelevant:** Deciding what information is pertinent to the situation at hand. *Example:* Deciding that the fact that someone's stepfather died of a heart attack is irrelevant to the person's *physical risk factors* for a heart attack.
- **Recognizing inconsistencies:** Realizing when there are contradictions within the presented information. *Example:* Noting that a child's injuries were unlikely to have happened in the way the parents describe.
- **Distinguishing normal from abnormal and identifying signs and symptoms (pieces of information that prompt you to suspect a**

problem): *Example:* Recognizing that a normally slightly wheezy asthmatic is now wheezing more than usual.

- **Clustering related information:** Putting together pieces of data that seem as though they should go together to get a beginning picture of patterns. *Example:* Putting together complaints of *poor appetite* and *difficulty preparing meals* and *depression.*
- **Identifying patterns:** Interpreting what patterns are suggested by the information you clustered together. *Example:* Considering the information above and deciding that there is a pattern of nutritional problems.
- **Identifying missing information:** Recognizing what pieces of information (data) are missing and finding the missing pieces. *Example:* Questioning the person above about food intake and checking for weight loss.
- **Drawing valid conclusions based on evidence:** Making deductions that follow logically. *Example:* In the above case, if there is evidence of weight loss, deciding that the person isn't eating enough because of the depression and inability to prepare meals.
- **Identifying several different conclusions:** Making sure all likely conclusions are considered. *Example:* Considering whether the weight loss above could be a sign of a more severe problem, such as *cancer,* or some other problem that should be evaluated by a physician.
- **Identifying underlying cause:** Deciding the main causes for a problem. *Example:* Deciding depression is a causative factor for the nutritional problem above.
- **Setting priorities:** Differentiating between problems needing immediate attention and those needing subsequent action. *Example:* Deciding that if the depression is resolved—perhaps by referring the problem to a doctor who could prescribe an antidepressant—the problem of not eating may be more readily addressed.
- **Evaluating and correcting our thinking:** Double-checking ourselves to make sure we've correctly accomplished the above skills and making required changes. *Example:* Realizing we were unsure about the reliability of the above person's family and double-checking to be sure the family is visiting every other day.

Did you find yourself noticing that some of the skills are things you already do without realizing it? Are you wondering, What's the point of addressing skills that seem like they should be automatic? The point is, you may do these automatically in familiar situations, but if you're *unaware* of what you're doing, it will be more difficult to transfer these skills to *new* situations. Remember the following rule.

■   **Rule: Critical thinking is contextual** (it happens within a set of circumstances for a specific purpose). Critical thinking skills require knowledge and experience and must be mastered *within each different context.*

In Chapter 5 you'll have the opportunity to practice key critical thinking skills by considering scenarios based on real nursing situations.

DEVELOPING CHARACTER, ACQUIRING KNOWLEDGE AND SKILLS

In summary, improving your thinking requires you to do three things:

1. **Develop a critical thinking character.** Hold yourself to high standards and make a commitment to develop critical thinking characteristics. Learn how to give and take feedback. To improve, we must get through the negative aspects of criticism.

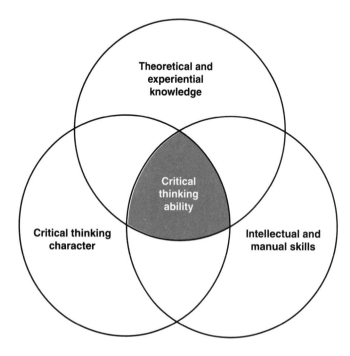

FIGURE 2–1

Critical thinking ability depends on having (1) critical thinking character (a commitment to developing critical thinking characteristics, attitudes, and dispositions), (2) theoretical and experiential knowledge (what to do, when and why you do it), and (3) intellectual and manual skills (critical thinking and psychomotor skills).

2. **Take responsibility and get actively involved.** Seek out learning resources and experiences that help you acquire the theoretical and experiential knowledge needed to think critically.
3. **Practice intellectual and manual skills in the context of how you'll use them.** Practicing intellectual skills such as assessing systematically and comprehensively helps make critical thinking more automatic. Also remember that until you master manual skills, for example, taking blood pressures, much of your brain power will go toward thinking about those types of skills, making it tougher to concentrate on *intellectual skills.*

Figure 2–1 provides a visual perspective of what's required to develop critical thinking ability.

OTHER PERSPECTIVES

"A good example has twice the value of good advice."   —Unknown

CRITICAL MOMENTS

How Ambiguous Can You Be?

Acceptance of ambiguity is often listed as a critical thinking characteristic. And certainly it's important to understand that sometimes there is, as the saying goes, "no black or white." A key point to be made, however, is that you need to ask, How much ambiguity is acceptable? For example, if you were sick, would you be happy with an ambiguous diagnosis or would you want it to be specific?

Picture This

When you're trying to understand, explain, or remember something, try drawing pictures, diagrams, or graphs. Our brains usually do better with pictures than words. For example, which of the ways of expressing percentages provided below is easiest for you to *understand?*

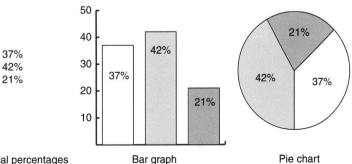

Numerical percentages   Bar graph   Pie chart

KEY POINTS

- Improved thinking requires gaining insight into what critical thinking is, acquiring instruction and feedback, and consciously practicing to improve.

- Gaining an awareness of your personal style—how and why you think and learn the way you do—is an excellent starting point for improving thinking.

- Each of us is responsible for connecting with our preferred styles and mastering strategies that can help us think and learn effectively in our *own* way.

- Connecting with your own particular personality type helps you gain insight into how and why you think the way you do. Understanding personality types different from your own helps you realize how and why *others* think the way *they* do. Boxes 2–1 and 2–2 (pages 28 and 29) summarize two different and complementary ways of describing personality type.

- Our ability to think well varies, depending on personal factors and circumstances that might be evident at the time. Table 2–1 (page 30) lists factors influencing critical thinking.

- Common habits creating barriers to critical thinking include *mine-is-better, choosing-only-one, face-saving, resistance to change, conformity, stereotyping,* and *self-deception.*

- Steven Covey offers seven habits that can enhance critical thinking by helping us build positive interpersonal relationships (page 39).

- The term **goal** usually focuses on **stating intent** (what you aim to do); the term **outcome** focuses on **describing results** (what actually gets accomplished from other people's perspectives). Outcomes are *specific results* that will be observed when your goal is achieved.

- Goals, because they focus on *intent,* may be vague, lofty, and unrealistic. Identifying *spe-*

cific, observable expected outcomes helps you be realistic and focused from the start.

- Outcomes should be (1) **well reasoned** (e.g., they should be realistic, considering the key players capabilities and available time and resources) and (2) **clearly stated** in terms that describe the results that will be observed when the outcomes are reached.

- Critical thinking requires that we develop strategies to help us communicate effectively (page 33 provides communication strategies).

- Page 43 outlines nine key questions you need to ask to help you determine your approach to critical thinking in any situation.

- Logic provides a foundation for critical thinking. It's the safest and most reliable strategy for problem solving.

- Using intuition as a guide to look for evidence is an effective strategy. Before you act on intuition alone, *however*—before you act on gut feelings that aren't supported by evidence—be sure your actions won't cause harm.

- Trial and error, or trying several solutions until one that works is found, is a risky but sometimes necessary approach to problem solving.

- Critical thinking is contextual (it happens within a set of circumstances for a specific purpose).

- Critical thinking skills require theoretical and experiential knowledge and must be mastered *within each different context.*

- Improving your thinking requires that you (1) hold yourself to high standards and make a commitment to develop critical thinking characteristics, attitudes, and dispositions, (2) take responsibility and get actively involved in finding learning resources and experiences, and (3) practice intellectual and manual skills in the context of how you'll use them.

CRITICAL THINKING EXERCISES

1. Using your own words and giving an example (or examples), explain how the terms *goal* and *outcome* are related.*

2. Think of an outcome that you'd like to achieve 6 months from now; then apply the nine key critical thinking questions in Box 2–5 to achieve your outcome.

3. How would your approach to critical thinking change in the following two situations?*
   a. You want your committee to produce a number of creative ideas to be evaluated at a later time.

   b. You want your committee to develop a policy for managing post-operative complications.

4. Arranging information into related patterns helps you remember better. Rearrange the following numbers into a pattern that helps you remember them:
   992887656780898

5. One of the fundamental skills to be acquired when learning to think critically is *identifying assumptions*—recognizing things you've taken for granted without realizing it. Answer the following riddle and then check the response on page 239 to see what assumptions you made. Think of a question you could have asked that may have helped you avoid making the assumptions.*

---

*An example response for this exercise can be found in the Response Key at the back of the book beginning on page 239.

▨ **Riddle:** Jack and Jill were found dead in a small puddle of water, surrounded by pieces of broken glass. There was no blood. What happened?

6. Respond to the following from the prechapter self-test:
    a. Explain the relationship between identifying outcomes and critical thinking.*
    b. Give five strategies that enhance critical thinking and provide reasons why the strategies work.*
    c. Explain why developing effective interpersonal and communication skills is essential to critical thinking.*
    d. Identify the roles of logic, intuition, and trial and error in critical thinking.*
    e. Describe at least five critical thinking skills you'd like to improve.
    f. Explain the relationship between critical thinking ability and developing character, knowledge, and skills.*

---

*An example response for this exercise can be found in the Response Key at the back of the book beginning on page 239.

3

Critical Thinking in Nursing: An Overview

This chapter at a glance . . .

Read the Learning Outcomes listed below and decide if you can readily achieve each one. If you can, you don't need to read this chapter and can go on to Chapter 4. Don't be concerned if you can't achieve any of the outcomes at this time. We'll come back to these outcomes later in the chapter, in Critical Thinking Exercises.

LEARNING OUTCOMES

After completing this chapter, you should be able to:

- Describe what critical thinking in nursing means to you in relation to the descriptions of critical thinking listed on pages 58 to 60.

- Name two major goals of nursing and discuss their implications for critical thinking.

- Describe what is meant by outcome-focused, data-driven, evidence-based care.

- Compare and contrast the *Diagnose and Treat* and the *Predict, Prevent, and Manage* approaches to health care delivery.

- Describe your responsibilities related to diagnosis and management of medical and nursing problems.

- Explain the role of ethics codes and national and facility standards and guidelines in making decisions.

- Identify a system to determine immediate priorities.

- Develop a personal plan to help you develop sound clinical judgment.

ABSTRACT

This is the first of two chapters focusing on how to think critically in the context of six common nursing concerns: clinical reasoning (clinical judgment), moral and ethical reasoning, nursing research, teaching others, teaching ourselves, and test taking. It starts by taking an in-depth look at the question, What is critical thinking in nursing? and addressing differences between novice and expert thinking. It then gives an overview of changes in health care affecting how nurses think. The remainder of the chapter is devoted to helping you develop the clinical reasoning skills required to succeed in today's challenging health care setting.

WHAT IS CRITICAL THINKING IN NURSING?

This section (Chapters 3 and 4) addresses critical thinking in six common nursing situations: reasoning in the clinical setting (clinical judgment), moral and ethical reasoning, nursing research, teaching others, teaching ourselves, and test taking. To keep the length of the chapters manageable—to avoid asking you to do too much at one time—content is divided into two chapters. This chapter provides an overview of critical thinking in nursing and focuses on the importance of developing clinical reasoning skills (clinical judgment). Chapter 4 focuses on moral and ethical reasoning, nursing research, teaching ourselves, teaching others, and test taking.

Applied Definition

Critical thinking is a complex process that can be described in different ways. Let's look at some of the different ways nurses describe critical thinking, starting with the applied definition from Chapter 1.

Critical thinking in nursing:
- Entails purposeful, outcome-directed (results-oriented) thinking.
- Is driven by patient, family, and community needs.
- Is based on principles of nursing process and scientific method.
- Requires specific knowledge, skills, and experience.
- Is guided by professional standards and ethics codes.
- Requires strategies that maximize human potential (e.g., using individual strengths) and compensate for problems created by hu-

man nature (e.g., the powerful influence of personal perspectives, values, and beliefs).

- Is constantly reevaluating, self-correcting, and striving to improve.

Other Ways Nurses Describe It

To many nurses, critical thinking means simply *good problem solving.* While certainly, problem-solving skills are required for critical thinking, you need a broader view of critical thinking to succeed in today's competitive workplace. You can't be satisfied with just having a "problem-solving mentality." You also need a sincere desire to improve—to find ways to broaden your knowledge and skills and to make current practices more efficient and effective, or you aren't thinking critically.

Joan Jenks, nursing faculty at Thomas Jefferson University in Philadelphia, says this about critical thinking: "Thinking critically involves paying attention to how one is thinking as nursing care is accomplished. Nurses should ask themselves questions like, *What are my assumptions in this situation? Are they accurate? What additional information do I need? How can I look at this situation in a different way?* This kind of thinking can occur while doing, or it can occur after doing. The important point is that nurses observe how thinking occurs and how effective it is. Critical thinking following doing is called *reflective thinking.* Thinking while doing is called *thinking in action.*"[1]

Another way to describe critical thinking is *a commitment to look for the best way, based on the most current research and practice findings,* for example, the best way to manage pain in a specific person or for a specific health problem. Figure 3–1 shows how critical thinking in nursing constantly strives to improve by focusing on two key questions: (1) What are the outcomes? and (2) How could we achieve these outcomes more efficiently?

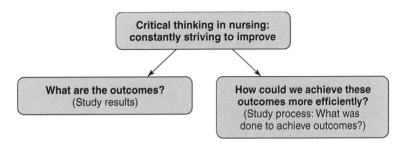

FIGURE 3–1

Goals of Nursing and Their Implications

To understand nursing's critical thinking, let's consider the questions, What are the goals of nursing (what do nurses aim to do)? and What are the implications of these goals?

Broadly speaking, nurses seek to accomplish two major goals in a humanistic, cost-effective, and timely way:

1. To help people avoid illness and its complications.
2. To help people gain an optimum level of independence and sense of well-being, regardless of health state (in cases of terminal illness the goal of dying comfortably is also appropriate).

So, what are the implications of these goals? Three major implications follow:

1. Because the conclusions and decisions we as nurses make *affect people's lives,* our thinking must be guided by sound reasoning—precise, disciplined thinking that promotes accuracy and depth of data collection and seeks to clearly identify the issues at hand.
2. Because we're committed to giving humanistic care, we must seek to help people within the context of *their* value systems—value systems that may be different from our own. We need to be aware of the *moral and ethical dimensions* of our thinking: We face situations that require making decisions about when to withhold judgment and when to speak up and say, No, that's wrong.
3. Because we're committed to achieving these goals in a cost-effective, timely fashion, we must constantly seek to improve both our personal ability to give nursing care *and* the overall efficiency of health care delivery.

Having made the above points, let's continue to look more closely at nursing's critical thinking, beginning with a discussion of how novice thinking differs from that of the expert. If we're aware of the differences, we can set realistic goals for developing critical thinking ability.

NOVICE THINKING VERSUS EXPERT THINKING

Consider the following scenario:

Scenario

A car hits a young man riding his bicycle in the park. Thrown 60 feet, he lies motionless. Within minutes two park rangers arrive. They put on latex gloves and begin to assess his injuries. An ambulance pulls up and one ranger yells, "We'll need intubation equipment!" A woman, out for a walk, looks on from a distance. A second woman, biking, comes upon the scene. Here's how the conversation goes:

First woman: This is terrible. I wish the ambulance had gotten here sooner.

Biking woman: Oh?

First woman: Yes. He was thrown at least 50 feet. If the ambulance had arrived sooner, they could have done more. I can't believe these two rangers didn't start resuscitation right away. They waited for this ambulance . . . they should have been breathing for him.

Biking woman: These rangers look like they know what they're doing. They would have started resuscitation if he needed it. This young man has been thrown so far, I'm sure they're concerned about spinal cord injuries. If they tilt his head back to start respirations, they risk severing his spinal cord—they don't want to do that unless it's absolutely necessary.

The above is a true story. I was the biking woman. As I talked more with the first woman, I learned she was a student nurse. She thanked me for pointing out something she hadn't thought about. After it was all over, I realized our conversation demonstrated a common difference between expert and novice thinking: the student nurse felt a need to *act* immediately. As an experienced nurse, I remembered the importance of *assessing* before acting.

We're all novices at one time or another. We all know what it's like to be new at something and watch an experienced professional and wonder, Will *I* ever know this much? And, almost always, with time and commitment, we soon find ourselves helping someone *else* who looks at *us* and thinks, Will *I* ever know this much?

To help you gain insight into novice thinking and expert thinking, study Table 3–1, which compares the two: If you're a novice, determine some things you can do to enhance your ability to think critically; if you're an expert, decide how you can help a novice.

TABLE 3–1	**Novice Thinking Compared With Expert Thinking**

The depth and breadth of expert knowledge, largely gained from opportunities to apply theory *in real situations,* greatly enhance critical thinking ability.

NOVICE NURSES	EXPERT NURSES
• Knowledge is organized as separate facts. Must rely heavily on resources (texts, notes, preceptors). Lack knowledge gained from actually doing (e.g., listening to breath sounds).	• Knowledge is highly organized and structured, making recall of information easier. Have a large storehouse of experiential knowledge (e.g., what abnormal breath sounds sound like, what subtle changes look like).
• Focus so much on *actions,* they tend to forget to *assess* before acting.	• *Assess* and think things through before *acting.*
• Need clear cut rules.	• Know when to bend the rules.
• Are often hampered by unawareness of resources.	• Are aware of resources and how to use them.
• Are often hindered by anxiety and lack of self-confidence.	• Are usually more self-confident, less anxious, and therefore more focused.
• Must be able to rely on step-by-step procedures. Tend to focus more on *procedures* than on the *patient response* to the procedure.	• Know when it's safe to skip steps or do two steps together. Are able to focus on both the parts (the procedures) and the whole (the patient response).
• Become uncomfortable if patient needs preclude performing procedures exactly as they were learned.	• Comfortable with rethinking procedure if patient needs require modification of the procedure.
• Have limited knowledge of suspected problems; therefore, they question and collect data more superficially.	• Have a better idea of suspected problems, allowing them to question more deeply and collect more relevant and in depth data.
• Tend to follow standards and policies by rote.	• Analyze standards and policies, looking for ways to improve them.
• Learn more readily when matched with a supportive, knowledgeable preceptor or mentor.	• Are challenged by novices' questions, clarifying their own thinking when teaching novices.

OTHER PERSPECTIVES

On Differences between Novices and Experts

"There is an accumulation of evidence that expert problem solving . . . is dependent on (1) a wealth of prior specific experiences that can be used in routine solution of problems by pattern recognition . . . and (2) elaborate conceptual knowledge applicable to the occasional problematic situation. . . . The main difference between expert clinicians and students is that experts generate better hypotheses (from the beginning, they have better hunches about what the problems may be)."[2]

–Dr. Geoffrey Norman

"In Japan we have the phrase shoshin, which means 'beginner's mind.' This does not mean a closed mind but actually an empty mind and a ready mind. If your mind is empty, it is always ready for anything. It is open to everything. In the beginners' mind, there are many possibilities; in the expert's mind there are few."

–Shunryu Suzuki, author of Zen Mind, Beginner's Mind

So now we've defined critical thinking in nursing and compared novice and expert thinking. Before going on to look at nursing process and clinical reasoning, let's look at some changes in health care delivery—changes you need to be aware of because of their profound influence on how we as nurses think.

A NEW MIND-SET FOR A NEW MILLENNIUM

A "new mind-set" is almost an oxymoron (a figure of speech with contradictory ideas) when it comes to critical thinking. Being a critical thinker requires us to *avoid* having a mind-set. We must keep an open mind that constantly questions the status quo. However, as a whole, we do have a new mind-set. And we must understand it to be able to think independently and critically in the real practice world. As you read this section, remember the importance of understanding the mind-set while challenging the status quo, looking for better ways.

Let's start by looking at how care delivery has shifted to a predictive model, a more proactive approach that prevents problems and maximizes health and independence.

SHIFT TO A PREDICTIVE MODEL

We're no longer satisfied with a *diagnose and treat* (DT) approach to health care—it implies that we wait for evidence of problems before beginning treatment. A DT approach is strong on *treating* problems but weak on *preventing* problems and their likely complications. Thanks to research, we now use a *predictive model*. We can *predict* who is at risk for certain problems and, if needed, begin an "aggressive prevention plan," which may include "treatment." Think about these examples:

- We may give an influenza vaccine to someone who has chronic lung disease and *also* vaccinate his entire family, thus reducing his risk of coming in contact with the influenza virus.
- In hip, back, and neck surgery, we routinely "treat to prevent" the potential complication of embolus (clot) formation. We apply pulsating antiemboli stockings and give anticoagulants.
- For those with significant exposure to the AIDS virus, treatment begins before we have evidence of the virus in the blood.
- Sometimes taking an antihistamine for a week *before* allergy season can make a significant difference in allergic response.

A predictive model is based on clinical studies. We now know that recovery from many problems follows an orderly pattern along predictable milestones. When patients fail to achieve a specific milestone, for example, if someone who has had open heart surgery isn't able to breath on his own within 24 hours of surgery, a multidisciplinary team evaluates whether there are problems to be solved or resources needed to get him back on track. (The milestone in this case is that the person should be able to breathe on his own within 24 hours.)

Predict, Prevent, and Manage (PPM)

Focusing on prevention through *early* intervention using a predictive model requires predicting, preventing, and managing problems and their likely complications. In other words, you do two things:

1. **In the presence of known problems, you predict the most *likely* and *most dangerous* complications** and take immediate action to

(a) prevent them and (b) be prepared to manage them in case they can't be prevented. *Example:* In cardiac emergencies, after defibrillation, intravenous lidocaine may be given to prevent other ventricular dysrhythmias. Emergency drugs and intubation equipment are kept readily available to manage unavoidable complications.

2. **Whether problems are present or not, you look for evidence of** ***risk and causative factors*** (things we know cause problems or put people at risk for problems). You then aim to control these factors to prevent the problems themselves. *Example:* You're visiting a home to assess a newborn. As part of the assessment, you determine whether there are risks to the infant's safety (e.g., you check where the baby sleeps, whether the parents are aware of possible infant hazards, whether the home has been "child proofed"). If you identify risks to the baby's safety, you're responsible for making a plan to correct the situation. Failing to make such a plan may be considered negligence.

The PPM approach, focusing on risk and causative factors, helps us prevent problems, prioritize care, and contain cost. Consider the following example:

> *Example:* It's believed that infants with electrocardiograms (ECGs) showing prolonged QT segments may be at risk for sudden infant death syndrome (SIDS). You might ask, Does that mean ECGs should be done on every newborn? The response may be, It's not necessary or cost effective—what we *must* do is make sure that one is done on every *high-risk* newborn (e.g., premature or low-birth-weight infant).

Treating versus Managing

We hear a lot about treating versus managing. You may be asking, What's the difference between these two?

Managing implies that you do more than *treat.* For example, in the case of asthma, you don't just keep treating asthma attacks. You act proactively, monitoring the person when healthy and fine-tuning care to keep the patient as free as possible from symptoms.

OUTCOME-FOCUSED, DATA-DRIVEN, EVIDENCE-BASED CARE

More than ever, care today is focused on outcomes. From professional and economic perspectives, we must recognize the importance of being able to answer questions like:

- Exactly what are the expected outcomes (specifically what will be observed *in this client or group* to show the benefit of nursing care)?
- By when do you expect to achieve these outcomes?
- What data or evidence is there that indicates that you're likely to achieve these outcomes?

In the past, we had little data about outcomes so we simply hoped for results. Today, in many cases, we're able to focus on realistic achievable outcomes based on data from clinical studies. For example, research continues on outcomes of hypertension management, pneumonia management, and home care visits by nurses. These studies give us important information we can use to show the need for nursing care and choose treatment plans most likely to work. Prevention and treatment are driven by the data, or evidence, collected over a period of time about how we can achieve the best results.

Box 3–1 summarizes additional trends in health care delivery influencing how nurses think.

CRITICAL MOMENT

Dealing with the Elderly and Chronically Ill

When dealing with aging and chronically ill clients, be careful of the human tendency to make assumptions. The complexity of their health status often hides problems that might otherwise be quite obvious. For example, we had a 70-year-old man with chronic back pain. He complained of increasing pain for weeks before someone said, "Maybe it's not his back. Has anyone checked his kidneys?" Only then were kidney stones diagnosed.

BOX 3–1	Summary of Health Care Trends: Health Care in the New Millennium

- **Nurses Take on More Responsibilities.** From staff nurses to those with advanced education and certification, nurses continue to take on more responsibilities for both diagnosis and management of health problems. Furthering education to master essential knowledge and skills and being willing to broaden clinical skills and responsibilities are keys to success. By staying focused on desired outcomes, providing humanistic care, and promoting health and independence, nurses continue to demonstrate how essential they are to improving health and well-being.

- **More Concern for Care of the Elderly and Chronically Ill.** We have a large population of people who are living longer with illnesses and disabilities. This group has special needs we must meet to keep them as healthy and independent as possible. When this group gets *sick*, the problems are often more complex than usual because of preexisting problems (for example, someone with a fractured hip may also have diabetes, chronic lung disease, and heart problems).

- **Greater Concern for Meeting Cultural Needs.** We are more aware of the importance of assessing cultural influences such as beliefs, values, and spiritual orientation. Nursing* and health care organizations† mandate that we identify cultural needs that may affect how someone responds to a plan of care (for example, if someone who is Muslim wants his bed turned toward Mecca 5 times a day, this request must be respectfully accommodated).

- **Care Moves from Hospitals to Homes.** Nursing care and "hi tech" equipment that used to be managed in hospitals is now managed in homes. Nurses must have excellent assessment and interpersonal skills and learn to be flexible, resourceful, and practical in the home care environment.

- **Multidisciplinary Approaches.** Boundaries between health care professionals continue to be flexible and ever changing as we seek to work together with other disciplines to improve outcomes. No one succeeds in isolated performance.

- **Computer Use.** Computers make it possible to track information in ways that were impossible in the past. We have instant access to vast knowledge stores, databases, and decision-support systems. By touching a few computer keys we can readily find the latest studies on a given topic or learn about responses to various treatment regimens. With this information at our fingertips, care is more knowledge based and patient specific. As this type of information explodes, nurses must know how to find and *use* information as much as they must know how to *memorize* it (see Using Information Effectively, pages 225 to 229).

*American Nurses Association. (1991). *Position statement on cultural diversity in nursing practice.* Kansas City, MO: Author.

†Joint Commission on Accreditation of Healthcare Organizations. (1997). *Accreditation Manual for Hospitals.* Oakbrook Terrace, IL: Author. *Box continued on following page*

BOX 3-1	**Summary of Health Care Trends: Health Care in the New Millennium** *Continued*

- **Refinement of Critical Paths‡ and Protocols.** Critical paths (standard multidisciplinary plans used to predict and determine appropriate care for specific problems) are constantly being refined and improved (see example, page 257). As we continue to track treatment and outcome data, we have more evidence-based protocols. For example, if you have asthma, you'll be more likely to receive specific treatment that's based on what studies show works best in most situations. As nurses, we continue to be responsible for thinking critically, recognizing when situations *vary* from the norm, and acting accordingly. For example, you may need to present a case for additional care or "stop everything" and call for multidisciplinary reevaluation.

- **Identification of Benchmarks and Best Practices.** National studies comparing regional protocols and guidelines help us to identify benchmarks and best practices (ways specific problems are best managed from an outcome and cost perspective). In other words, we'll see more consensus about the best ways to prevent and manage common problems.

- **Case Management.** Case management—the use of collaborative approaches to ensure that the best available resources are used to reach outcomes efficiently—promotes quality. This approach is firmly grounded in prevention and early intervention. Today all nurses are expected to be "case managers," closely monitoring progress toward outcomes to detect variances in care (a *variance in care* is when a patient isn't progressing toward outcomes in the expected time frame—for example, if someone has surgery and is expected to get out of bed on the first day after surgery but is unable to do so, it's considered a *variance in care*, which needs further evaluation).

- **Services Driven by Consumer and Community Needs.** Health care organizations aiming to succeed recognize that they must compete for their clients' dollars—services must be driven by consumer needs and customer satisfaction. Insurance companies and consumers alike want to know that they are getting the best value for their dollar. We must continually examine what people perceive as "value." For example, one person may value low cost over convenience, while another may be more concerned with convenience than cost. We can no longer approach health care delivery with a "one size fits all" mentality. We must ask questions like, What are the physical, developmental, cultural, and socioeconomic needs of this specific patient or group? How can we add value to what we offer? and What can we do to improve customer satisfaction? Today's nurses must be adept at skills required for customer satisfaction (for example, see Developing Empowered Partnerships, Dealing with Complaints, Managing Conflict Constructively, Communicating Bad News, in Chapter 6).

‡Also known as clinical pathways and CareMaps™. See page 257 for an example.

BOX 3–1	**Summary of Health Care Trends: Health Care in the New Millennium** *Continued*

- **Managed Care.** The goal of managed care is to furnish services within a group of providers who network to provide quality care in the most cost-effective manner. Nurses, physicians, and therapists working in a managed care environment are challenged to deliver the highest standard of care with the best value. By continuing to track patient outcomes and provide evidence for what really works in the long run, we can build cases for reimbursement for essential diagnostic and treatment modalities.
- **Wellness Centers, Holistic and Alternative Therapies.** As people live longer with more chronic problems, we continue to focus more on preventive health care. We realize the value of keeping people healthy and triggering the body's natural healing powers through holistic and alternative therapies (e.g., diet, exercise, acupuncture, and stress reduction through meditation and aroma therapy). We have entire communities coming together to focus on wellness (for example, Celebration City near Orlando, Florida). The Office of Alternative Medicines lists over 60 alternative health care practices (see their Web page at *http://altmed.od.nih.gov*).
- **Direct Advertising to Consumers Who Must Make Educated Choices.** Carefully scripted ads encourage consumers to ask for specific drugs (e.g., "Ask your doctor about Zocor") or to come to certain facilities (e.g., "If you have a wound that doesn't heal, come to our wound care center."). Nurses are called on to help consumers at both ends of the "knowledge spectrum," from those who are illiterate to those who travel the Internet, becoming experts on the latest information on their problems.

CRITICAL THINKING EXERCISES

1. Get out a piece of paper and make two columns. On the left, list the key points of the applied critical thinking definition on page 58. On the right, write your own interpretation of what each key point implies about what you need to do to think critically in nursing.

2. Write a few statements that address the implications of the following Critical Moment in relation to developing critical thinking skills.*

    CRITICAL MOMENT

   Acquiring Knowledge and Skills
   Many nurses focus on acquiring *skills* (they want to begin *doing* things as soon as possible). However, knowledge usually comes before skills: To truly master a skill, you must first master the *facts* you must know to perform the skill safely and effectively. To help you learn by *doing* in a safe environment, seek out simulated exercises.

3. Study Table 3–1, page 62 (Novice Thinking Compared with Expert Thinking). Write a paragraph or two about how you think in relation to the descriptions in this table.

4. What's wrong with this "picture" (the following scenario)?*

   Scenario
   Mr. Gimenez, a debilitated diabetic, is seen at home every other day by a nurse, who checks a healing incision. Mr. Gimenez has been looking for an assistive device to attach to the toilet to help him get up and down. When he asks the visiting nurse if she knows where she can find such a device, the nurse replies, "I'm sorry. I know what you mean, but I don't know where you get them."

---

*An example response for this exercise can be found in the Response Key at the back of the book beginning on page 239.

5. Using your own words and giving examples, explain how you use a predict, prevent, and manage approach to health care delivery.*

6. Respond to the following from the prechapter self-test.
    a. Describe what critical thinking in nursing means to you in relation to the descriptions of critical thinking listed on pages 58 to 60.
    b. Name two major goals of nursing and discuss their implications for critical thinking.*
    c. Describe what is meant by outcome-focused, data-driven, evidence-based care.*
    d. Compare and contrast the *Diagnose and Treat* and the *Predict, Prevent, and Manage* approaches to health care delivery.*

A CHANGING NURSING PROCESS

Use of the nursing process summarized in Box 3–2 is required by national practice standards,† provides a basis for critical thinking in nursing. Yet how we teach and use it is changing.

Less Linear, More Dynamic

In the past the nursing process was viewed as being a rigid, linear method that started with *assessment* and ended with *evaluation.* Now we realize that it's dynamic and that nurses move back and forth within the steps. Here are two examples:

1. You're performing an *assessment* (step 1) and haven't yet *identified the problems* (step 2). You may decide it's appropriate to help the person get into a more comfortable position (*perform an intervention,* step 4) before you complete a comprehensive *assessment* (step 1). Once immediate problems are handled, you go on to complete the steps of the nursing process to make sure you don't miss anything.

---

*An example response for this exercise can be found in the Response Key at the back of the book beginning on page 240.

†American Nurses Association. (1991). *Standards of Clinical Practice.* Washington, DC: Author, and Canadian Nurses Association. (1987). *Standards for Nursing Practice.* Ottawa, Canada: Author.

BOX 3–2	**Nursing Process As a Tool for Critical Thinking**

1. **Assessment.** Continuously and deliberately collecting and recording data to provide the information required to:
   - Anticipate, detect, prevent, manage, or eliminate health problems.
   - Identify ways of helping people obtain optimum wellness and independence.
   - Evaluate efficiency of care delivery.
2. **Diagnosis.** Analyzing data, putting related information together, drawing conclusions, and identifying:
   - Actual and potential health problems.
   - Underlying risk factors and causes of the health problems.
   - Resources and strengths.
   - Health states that are satisfactory but could be improved.
3. **Planning.** Determining specific desired outcomes and interventions by predicting responses. The interventions are designed to:
   - Detect, prevent, and manage health problems.
   - Promote optimum wellness and independence.
   - Achieve the desired outcomes in a timely, cost-effective way.
4. **Implementation.** Putting the plan into action by:
   - Assessing readiness to perform interventions
   - Performing interventions, then reassessing to determine initial responses.
   - Making immediate changes as needed.
   - Keeping records to monitor progress.
5. **Evaluation.** Determining whether the expected outcomes have been met; modifying or terminating the plan as appropriate; planning for ongoing continuous assessment and improvement.

2. Sometimes you deal with standard plans that have already done much of the work of steps 2 and 3 (*planning and implementation*) for you. Instead of having to create a plan "from scratch," you must decide whether the standard plan *is appropriate* for each particular patient. Standard plans don't *think* for you. You must think independently, *applying principles* of nursing process like assessing before acting and predicting responses to interventions before acting.

Figure 3–2 shows how a critical thinker uses a more proactive, dynamic approach to nursing process than a noncritical thinker uses.

While the nursing process is certainly more dynamic than we first understood, it's important to remember the following rule:

■ **Rule**
- **Experts often use the nursing process in a very dynamic way because they know what steps can be safely skipped or delayed.** They also know when situations warrant a rigorous, comprehensive, step-by-step approach.
- **Beginners often need to follow the steps more rigidly, carefully reflecting on each step.** Because of their inexperience, they take more risks when skipping or delaying steps.

Is the Care Plan Dead?

As critical paths and standard plans have replaced personally developed care plans, some nurses have begun to say things like, nursing process and care planning is dead. However, the care plan is alive and well. It's only changed. Standards in most health care organizations—from hospitals to nursing homes—mandate that clients have a recorded plan of care that demonstrates that their specific needs and problems are being addressed.

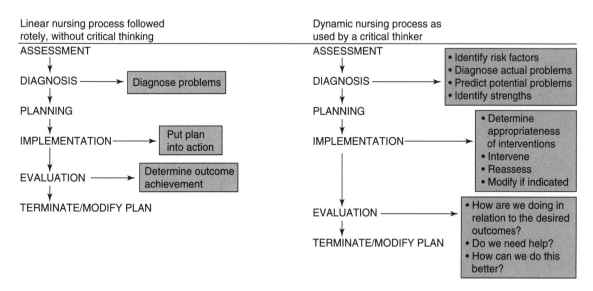

FIGURE 3-2

How a noncritical thinker might use the nursing process compared with how a critical thinker might use the nursing process, focusing on the diagnosis, implementation, and evaluation stages.

Today, you may not find the care plan in one place. Rather, parts of the plan may be addressed in different places of the chart (the nursing assessment may be in one place, a critical path delineating interventions in another, an individual plan in another, and so on). For this reason, you *must* be familiar with principles of nursing process and care planning to be able to *know* whether the plan of care is sufficiently documented. Whether you're developing a plan yourself or using standard plans, remember the following rule:

▧ **Rule:** Care plans include the following components:
- Expected outcomes
- Actual and potential problems, which must be addressed to achieve the overall outcomes
- Specific interventions designed to achieve the outcomes
- Evaluation statements (progress notes)

What Do Nurses Diagnose?

Another major change in how we use nursing process is in step 2, diagnosis. We have moved from "nurses diagnose and treat only nursing diagnoses" to "nurses diagnose and manage various problems, depending on their knowledge, expertise, and qualifications." For example, advanced practice nurses (APN) and other specially trained nurses may diagnose or manage problems that used to be managed only by physicians.

So then, how do you know when you're accountable for diagnosing and managing a problem? This is a tough question for beginning nurses. It often takes varied experiences thinking *in the clinical setting* for the concept of accountability for diagnosis and management to come alive. However, let's begin by considering the implications of the terms in the following rule:

▧ **Rule:** The terms *diagnose* and *diagnosis* have legal implications. They imply that there's a specific problem that requires management by a qualified expert.
- If you make a diagnosis, it means that you accept accountability for accurately naming and managing the problem independently.
- If you treat a problem or allow a problem to persist without ensuring that the correct diagnosis has been made, you may cause harm and be accused of negligence.
- You're accountable for detecting, identifying, or recognizing signs and symptoms that may indicate problems beyond your expertise.

Example: Bedside nurses aren't qualified or accountable for diagnosing and managing pneumonia independently. **However, they *are* accountable for:**

- Detecting and reporting *signs and symptoms* of pneumonia (e.g., fever, productive cough, malaise).
- Diagnosing and managing *risk factors* for pneumonia, for example, weak breathing efforts due to surgical pain, spinal cord injury, or disease (in complicated cases, these risk factors may require medical management).
- Diagnosing and managing *human responses* to pneumonia (e.g., problems caused by pneumonia, such as mobility and nutritional problems).

Nursing Responsibilities Related to Diagnosis

Understanding *conceptually* the types of problems that nurses focus on is an important step toward understanding your responsibilities related to diagnosis and management of health problems. Following are examples of the types of problems that nurses commonly manage:

- **Risks for injury.** At every patient encounter, nurses are responsible for detecting risks for injury and intervening accordingly. For example, the following are common nursing concerns:
  - Preventing falls
  - Preventing skin breakdown
  - Controlling risks for violence
  - Controlling risks for infection
- **Knowledge deficits.** Nurses are often accountable for ensuring that patients or their caregivers have the knowledge required to manage their own health. For example, diabetic teaching is a nursing responsibility.
- **Promoting comfort and managing pain.** Nurses play a major role in promoting comfort and managing pain through both medical and holistic therapies.
- **Problems that impede ability to be independent and live a healthy lifestyle.** For example, managing problems with performing activities of daily living (ADL) such as bathing and dressing is a nursing responsibility.
- **Tailoring of treatment and medication regimens for each individual.** Nurses are intimately involved in ensuring that overall regimens are as safe, effective, cost effective, and convenient as possible, considering the age, culture, religion, roles, occupation, and lifestyles of those involved.
- **Disease prevention and health promotion.** Nurses are concerned with preventing illness and promoting health by detecting and

managing risk factors for problems with nutrition, elimination, coping, rest, exercise, and so on.

- **Monitoring for changes in health status.** Because nurses are the ones who spend the most time with patients—the ones in the "front line" so to speak—they are concerned with detecting signs and symptoms of possible problems requiring medical (or other multidisciplinary) management. For example, in the case of surgery, you're responsible for recognizing and reporting signs of potential complications, such as excessive blood loss.

- **Human responses** (how individuals, families, or groups *respond* to health problems or life changes). For example, suppose a man has surgery for breast cancer. His human response, how he *responds* to his medical condition—whether he has problems with self-esteem, sexuality, or whatever—is a nursing concern. The following definition of nursing diagnosis addresses nursing responsibilities in relation to human responses:

  - **Nursing diagnosis:** A clinical judgment about an individual, family, or community response to actual or potential health problems and life processes. Nursing diagnoses provide the basis for selection of nursing interventions to achieve outcomes for which the nurse is accountable.[3]

Now that you have a conceptual idea of common nursing concerns, let's take a different approach to understanding what it is that nurses diagnose. Appendix E, page 264, shows diagnoses accepted for clinical testing by the North American Nursing Diagnosis Association (NANDA). **You aren't expected to know every diagnosis on the list.** Rather, you need to find out which of the diagnoses have been accepted for use by your school or facility. Some schools and facilities have made significant improvements in identifying nursing problems by using NANDA-recommended diagnostic labels, while others focus more on nursing responsibilities in the context of medical problems and use of critical paths.

Box 3–3, page 77, shows nursing diagnoses commonly used by rehabilitation nurses. There are other diagnoses commonly used in other nursing specialties. As you study (or work in) different specialty practices, for example, pediatrics or maternity nursing, you need to check with experts, up-to-date texts, and policies and procedures to determine the types of problems you're expected to diagnose and manage.

BOX 3-3	**Diagnoses Commonly Identified in Rehabilitation Nursing**

Risk for injury
Activity intolerance
Impaired physical mobility
Colonic constipation
Reflex incontinence
Urinary retention
Feeding self-care deficit
Bathing or hygiene self-care deficit
Dressing and grooming self-care deficit
Toileting self-care deficit
Pressure ulcer

Pain
Knowledge deficit
Impaired swallowing
Impaired thought processes
Body image disturbance
Impaired verbal communication
Ineffective individual coping
Ineffective family coping
Caregiver role strain
Risk for disuse syndrome

Data from Association of Rehabilitation Nurses. (1995). *21 Rehabilitation nursing diagnoses: A guide to interventions and outcomes.* Glenview, IL: Author.

Box 3–4, pages 78 and 79, shows examples of common medical problems together with related complications. These are all common problems that nurses must know before graduating from nursing school. Whether you use nursing diagnoses or not, keep in mind the following rule:

▧ **Rule:** To be sure you detect both nursing and possible medical problems:
- Use a **nursing model** to collect data to be sure you detect nursing problems (see Boxes 3–5 and 3–6).
- Use a **body systems** approach to help you identify problems that may require medical management (see Figure 3–3). You use a body systems approach because medical diagnoses are usually related to problems with structure and function of **body organs or systems.**

 OTHER PERSPECTIVES

From Critical Pathways to Life Pathways
"The rehabilitation nurse's role is expanding. We now go beyond traditional, episodic case management to life management, beyond disease management to life care prevention: beyond critical pathways to life pathways." —*Terri Patterson, RN, MSN, CRRN President, LifeTrak Ltd.*

Text continues on page 82

BOX 3–4	**Common Complications**

Common medical diagnoses (in bold) *and their potential complications*

Angina/myocardial infarction
- Dysrhythmias
- Congestive heart failure/pulmonary edema
- Shock (cardiogenic, hypovolemic)
- Infarction, infarction extension
- Thrombi/emboli formation (e.g., pulmonary emboli, cerebrovascular accident)
- Hypoxemia
- Electrolyte imbalance
- Acid-base imbalance
- Pericarditis
- Cardiac tamponade
- Cardiac arrest

Asthma/chronic obstructive lung disease
- Hypoxemia
- Acid-base/electrolyte imbalance
- Respiratory failure
- Cardiac failure
- Infection

Diabetes
- Hyper/hypoglycemia
- Delayed wound healing
- Hypertension
- Eye problems (retinal hemorrhage)
- *See also* Angina/myocardial infarction

Fractures
- Bleeding
- Fracture displacement
- Thrombus/embolus formation
- Compromised circulation (pressure points, edema)
- Nerve compression
- Infection
- *See also* Skeletal traction/casts

Head trauma
- Increased intracranial pressure (secondary to bleeding or brain swelling)
- Respiratory depression
- Shock
- Hyper/hypothermia
- Coma

Hypertension
- Cerebrovascular accident
- Transient ischemic attacks (TIAs)
- Renal failure
- Hypertensive crisis
- *See also* Angina/myocardial infarction

Pneumonia
- Respiratory failure
- Sepsis/septic shock

Pulmonary embolus
- *See* Angina/myocardial infarction

Renal failure
- Fluid overload
- Hyperkalemia
- Electrolyte/acid-base imbalance
- Anemia
- *See also* Hypertension

Trauma
- *See* Anesthesia/surgical or invasive procedures

Urinary tract infection
- Septic shock

BOX 3–4	**Common Complications** *Continued*

Common treatment and diagnostic modalities (in bold) and their potential complications

Anesthesia/surgical or invasive procedures
  Bleeding/hypovolemia/shock
  Respiratory depression/atelectasis
  Urinary retention
  Fluid/electrolyte imbalances
  Thrombus/embolus formation
  Paralytic ileus
  Incisional complications (infection, poor
    healing, dehiscence/evisceration)
  Sepsis/septic shock
Cardiac catheterization
  Bleeding
  Thrombus/embolus formation
Chest tubes
  Hemo/pneumothorax
  Bleeding
  Atelectasis
  Chest tube malfunction/blockage
  Infection/sepsis
Foley catheter
  Infection/sepsis
  Catheter malfunction/blockage

Intravenous therapy
  Phlebitis/thrombophlebitis
  Infiltration/extravasation
  Fluid overload
  Infection/sepsis
  Bleeding
  Air embolism
Medications
  Adverse reactions (allergic response/
    exaggerated effects/side effects/drug
    interactions)
  Overdose/toxicity
Nasogastric suction
  Electrolyte imbalance
  Tube malfunction/blockage
  Aspiration
Skeletal traction/casts
  Poor bone alignment
  Bleeding/swelling
  Compromised circulation
  Nerve compression
  See also Fractures

From Alfaro-LeFevre, R. (1994). *Applying nursing process: A step-by-step guide* (3rd ed.). Philadelphia: J.B. Lippincott.

Summarized from Gordon, M. (1987). *Nursing diagnosis: Process and application.* New York: McGraw-Hill.

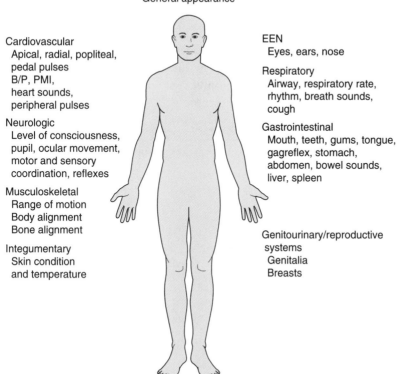

BODY SYSTEMS ASSESSMENT

General appearance

Cardiovascular
Apical, radial, popliteal, pedal pulses
B/P, PMI, heart sounds, peripheral pulses

Neurologic
Level of consciousness, pupil, ocular movement, motor and sensory coordination, reflexes

Musculoskeletal
Range of motion
Body alignment
Bone alignment

Integumentary
Skin condition and temperature

EEN
Eyes, ears, nose

Respiratory
Airway, respiratory rate, rhythm, breath sounds, cough

Gastrointestinal
Mouth, teeth, gums, tongue, gagreflex, stomach, abdomen, bowel sounds, liver, spleen

Genitourinary/reproductive systems
Genitalia
Breasts

FIGURE 3–3

Body systems assessment.

BOX 3–6	A Frequently Used Nursing Model: Human Response Patterns

Exchanging

Cardiac
Cerebral
Peripheral
Skin integrity
Oxygenation
Physical regulation
Nutrition
Elimination

Communicating

Read/write/understand English, other
   languages, impaired speech, other forms of
   communication

Relating

Relationships
Socialization

Valuing

Religious preference, important religious
   practices, spiritual concerns, cultural
   orientation, cultural practices

Choosing

Coping
Participation in health regimen
Judgment

Moving

Activity
Rest
Recreation
Environmental maintenance
Health maintenance
Self-care
Meaningfulness
Sensory perception

Perceiving

Self-concept
Meaningfulness
Sensory perception

Knowing

Current health problems
Health history
Current medications
Risk factors
Readiness to learn
Mental status
Memory

Feeling

Pain/discomfort
   associated/aggravating/alleviating factors
Emotional integrity/status

From Iyer, P.W., Taptich, B.J., and Bernocchi-Losey, D. (1991). *Nursing process and nursing diagnosis* (2nd ed., p. 51). Philadelphia: W.B. Saunders Co.

WHAT IS CLINICAL JUDGMENT?

The terms *clinical judgment, clinical reasoning,* and *critical thinking* are often used interchangeably. This section clarifies the relationship between these terms and discusses how to develop clinical judgment. Let's start by considering the rule below, which explains what clinical judgment means in the context of nursing practice.

■ **Rule:** Clinical judgment has two meanings:
1. **Nursing opinion(s)** made about a person's, family's, or group's health at a certain point in time.
2. **Nursing decisions** made about things like what to assess, what health data suggest, what to do first, and who should do it.

Keep in mind the following key points about clinical judgment:
 1. You use *clinical reasoning and critical thinking* to make clinical judgments.
 2. Clinical judgments (your nursing opinions) are extremely important because they guide nursing care.
 3. Ability to make clinical judgments depends on theoretical and experiential knowledge—for example, knowing what to look for, how to recognize when a patient's status is changing, and what to do about it.
 4. Using "sound clinical judgment" means drawing valid conclusions and then *acting appropriately* based on those conclusions. *Example:* Drawing the conclusion that you don't know enough to handle a specific problem and acting by consulting with a more experienced professional. Keep the following rule in mind:

■ **Rule:** In clinical judgment the term *clinical* implies that the judgment is made in the *clinical setting*—often a "thinking on your feet" type of thinking. However, clinical judgment also includes knowing when the situation requires more than "thinking on your feet," for example, knowing when the situation is so complex that you need to take your time or get additional opinions before drawing a conclusion.

Developing clinical judgment is perhaps one of the most important and challenging aspects of becoming a nurse. It's important because people's lives depend on it. It's challenging because thinking in the clinical setting is often fraught with more anxiety and risks than other situations.

For beginners, clinical reasoning is particularly challenging because it requires an ability to recall facts, put them together into a meaningful whole, and apply the information to the real world. For example, You note that someone is pale, sweaty, and has a rapid pulse. To use good clinical judgment, you need to be able to *recall* that these are possible symptoms of shock and that an immediate priority is to take a complete set of vital signs to further evaluate the patient's condition.

Being able to make effective clinical judgments comes from a "marriage" of theoretical and experiential knowledge—it requires that you apply what you know from class, readings, and simulation exercises to the real practice world. If you practice without theoretical knowledge, you're unlikely to make sound clinical judgments. If you have only theoretical knowledge, with little clinical experience, you're also unlikely to make sound clinical judgments.

SCOPE OF PRACTICE DECISIONS

A key aspect of developing clinical judgment is learning to make decisions about what actions are within your scope of practice. In other words, how do you know when you're qualified to render an opinion or perform a nursing action? Because laws and standards constantly change, several nursing boards have developed guides to help nurses make these types of decisions (see Fig. 3–4, page 84, an example guideline for students).

DECISION MAKING AND NURSING STANDARDS AND GUIDELINES

Critical thinking in nursing is guided by professional standards. Let's look at how decision making in nursing is influenced by broad and specific standards.

National practice standards provide broad standards that address how nurses are expected to plan and deliver care (see Appendix F, Standards for Practice, page 267). Each specialty organization (e.g., American Association of Critical-Care Nurses, Association of Rehabilitation Nurses, Association of Operating Room Nurses) has also developed its own standards for specialty practice.

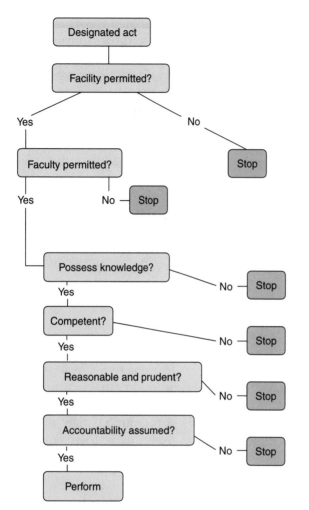

FIGURE 3–4

Model to aid student decision making. (Adapted from Pennsylvania State Board of Nursing Decision-making Model.)

Each facility has developed numerous specific standards and guidelines (standards of care, policies, protocols, procedures, care plans, and critical paths) that are intended to aid decision making in *specific* situations. The *Agency for Health Care Policy and Research* has also developed national practice guidelines for the care of some specific problems (see Box 3–7, page 85).

There are three questions to raise when making decisions about how to manage health problems:

1. Has this facility developed specific guidelines or policies for the care of this specific situation? For example, if you're caring for

someone with a mastectomy, you need to ask, Has this facility developed any type of guidelines for someone undergoing a mastectomy?

2. Are there national practice guidelines relating to this particular problem?

3. To what degree do these standards apply to my specific patient's situation?

Facility and national guidelines are valuable tools to help you make care decisions. However, you don't follow guidelines *blindly.* An essential part of decision making is using critical thinking to recognize when the situation at hand *differs* from the guide. You must carefully compare *your patient's data with the information presented in the guideline* and decide whether the guidelines are indeed applicable to your specific patient. For

BOX 3–7	**Examples of Practice Guidelines Available from the Agency for Health Care Policy and Research (AHCPR)***

- Acute low back problems
- Acute pain
- Benign prostatic hyperplasia
- Cancer screening
- Cardiac rehabilitation
- Cataracts in adults
- Colorectal cancer
- Sickle cell disease
- Depression
- Early HIV infection
- Heart failure

- Management of cancer pain
- Otitis media
- Post-stroke rehabilitation
- Pressure ulcers in adults: prediction and prevention
- Quality determinants of mammography
- Screening for Alzheimer's disease
- Smoking cessation
- Treatment of pressure ulcers
- Urinary incontinence

Want to Know More? Visit the AHCPR Web site at http://www.ahcpr.gov where you can read and download the latest guidelines. You can also contact the AHCPR Publications Clearinghouse, Box 8547, Silver Spring, MD 20907. Phone: 1-800-358-9295

*This is not a comprehensive list. Guidelines are available in several formats: *Clinical Practice Guidelines* and *Quick Reference Guides for Clinicians* are intended for health care providers; *Consumer Versions,* also available in Spanish, are intended for patients and family members.

example, suppose you're caring for someone who just had prostate surgery and the critical path for this problem states that on the second day the patient will get out of bed twice. However, on the second day, you assess the man and find he has chest discomfort. This finding is significant enough for you to question whether he should indeed get out of bed today: Could this man be suffering a complication such as myocardial infarction or pulmonary embolus? In this case, you need to report the symptoms and keep the man in bed until a physician or advanced practice nurse evaluates him.

OTHER PERSPECTIVES

Theoretical Pros and Cons of Critical Paths

As we continue to refine critical paths, David Nash, Associate Dean for Health Policy at Jefferson Medical College in Philadelphia, Pennsylvania, points out the following pros and cons[4]:

Pros	Cons
• Predictable expectations	• Still in early stages of development
• Clear progress markers	• Don't accommodate outliers (those with unusual problems and slow recovery)
• Allows treatment analysis along path	• Justifies curtailing services
• Provides standards to evaluate outcomes	• Risk of ethical hazards

HOW TO DEVELOP EFFECTIVE CLINICAL JUDGMENT

Developing clinical reasoning skills takes time. It also requires a commitment to study common health problems, seek out clinical experiences, and come prepared to the clinical setting. In Chapter 5, you'll have opportunities to practice skills that are essential to critical thinking and developing clinical judgment (e.g., drawing valid conclusions, setting priorities). For now, review Box 3–8, page 87, which answers the nine critical thinking questions from Chapter 2 in relation to clinical judgment. Once you've done that, consider the following strategies for developing effective clinical judgment.

| BOX 3–8 | **Clinical Judgment: Nine Key Questions** |

1. **What major outcomes (observable beneficial results) do we expect to see *in this particular person, family, or group* when the plan of care is terminated?**

   Example: The person will be discharged infection free, able to care for himself, 3 days after surgery.

   Outcomes may be addressed on a standard plan or you may have to develop these outcomes yourself.* Be sure that you check to make sure any predetermined outcomes in standard plans are *appropriate* to your patient's specific situation.

2. **What problems or issues *must* be addressed to achieve the major outcomes?** Answering this question will help you set priorities. You might be faced with a long list of actual or potential health problems. You need to narrow down your list to those that *must* be addressed.

3. **What are the circumstances?** *Who's* involved (e.g., child, adult, group)? How urgent are the problems (e.g., life-threatening, chronic)? What are the factors influencing their presentation (e.g., when, where, and how did the problems develop)? What are the patient's values, beliefs, and cultural influences?

4. **What knowledge is required?** Knowledge required includes problem-specific facts (e.g., how health problems usually present, how they're diagnosed, what their common causes and risk factors are, what common complications occur, and how these complications are prevented and managed); nursing process and related knowledge and skills (ethics, research, health assessment, communication, priority setting); related sciences (anatomy, physiology, pathophysiology, pharmacology, chemistry, physics, psychology, sociology). You must also be clearly aware of the circumstances, as addressed in No. 3 above.

5. **How much room is there for error?** In the clinical setting, there is usually minimal room for error. However, it depends on the health of the individual and risks of interventions. *Example:* In which of the following cases do you think you have more room for error?

   - You're trying to decide whether to give a healthy child a onetime dose of acetaminophen for heat rash without checking with the doctor.
   - You have a child who's been sick for 3 days with a fever and the mother wants to know if she should continue giving acetaminophen without checking with the doctor.

   If you thought *the first one* above, you're right. In the *second* case, the symptoms have continued for 3 days without a diagnosis. If you continue to give acetaminophen without checking with a physician, you might be masking symptoms of a problem requiring medical management.

*Chapter 5 gives practice exercises for developing outcomes.   *Box continued on following page*

BOX 3–8	**Clinical Judgment: Nine Key Questions** *Continued*

6. **How much time do I have?** Time frame for decision making depends on (a) the urgency of the problems (e.g., there's less time in life-threatening situations, such as cardiac arrest) and (b) the planned length of contact (e.g., if your patient will be hospitalized only for 2 days, you have to be realistic about what can be accomplished, and key decisions need to be made *early*).

7. **What resources can help me?** Human resources include clinical nurse educators, nursing faculty, preceptors, more experienced nurses, advance practice nurses, peers, librarians, and other health care professionals (pharmacists, nutritionists, physical therapists, physicians). The patient and family are also valuable resources (usually they know their own problems best). Other resources include texts, articles, other references, and computer data bases and decision-making support; national practice guidelines, facility documents (e.g., guidelines, policies, procedures, assessment forms).

8. **Whose perspectives must be considered?** The most significant perspective to consider is the patient's point of view. Other important perspectives include those of the family and significant others, caregivers, and relevant third parties (e.g., insurers).

9. **What's influencing my thinking?** Be sure you identify personal biases. Thinking may also be influenced by any of the factors listed in Table 2–1, Factors Influencing Critical Thinking (page 30).

TEN STRATEGIES FOR DEVELOPING CLINICAL JUDGMENT

1. **Until you have enough repeated experiences with diagnosis and management of commonly encountered health problems, keep references such as notes, texts, and pocket guides readily available.** Unless you have repeated experiences, you're unlikely to be able to recall the information you need to think and act appropriately.

   • **Learn terminology and concepts.** If you encounter words like *embolus*, *thrombus*, or *phlebitis* and you don't know what they mean, you'll be unable to understand and learn. Look up new terms and concepts *as you encounter them* and they'll soon become a part of your long-term memory. Learning the terms *in context* also helps you store information in related groups, rather than as isolated facts.

   • **Become familiar with normal findings before being concerned with abnormal findings** (e.g., lab values, physical assessment findings, disease progression, growth and development): Once you know what's *normal*, you'll readily recognize when you encounter information that is *outside the norm* (abnormal).

- **Always ask why.** Find out what theories or principles explain why *normal* findings occur and why *abnormal* findings occur.
- **Learn problem-specific facts.** You need to know how problems usually present (their signs and symptoms), what usually causes them, and how they're managed. For instance, if you're going to take care of someone who has a medical diagnosis of *diabetes* and a nursing diagnosis of *ineffective individual coping*, become familiar with the signs, symptoms, and common causes, complications, and management of these two problems before caring for the person. Box 3–9 provides questions you should ask to gain the facts you'll need to know to reason well in the clinical setting.

BOX 3–9	**Questions You Need To Answer to Gain Problem-Specific Knowledge Before Taking Care of Someone in the Clinical Setting**

1. What problems do I know or suspect my patient has?
2. What risk factors do I know or suspect my patient has?
3. What are the signs and symptoms of these problems?
4. What must I assess to determine the status of these signs, symptoms, and risk factors?
5. What are the usual causes of these problems?
6. What must I assess to determine the status of the *causes* of the problems?
7. How do these problems usually progress, and how are they managed?
8. How can these problems be prevented?
9. What could cause these problems to change, and in what way?
10. What are the signs and symptoms of potential complications of these problems and how will I monitor for these signs and symptoms?
11. How can I be prepared to manage potential complications if they should occur?
12. What medications and treatments are likely to be used, and why?
13. What medication-related or treatment-related problems might I encounter; how will I monitor to detect them; and how are they usually managed?
14. What cultural factors, values, or beliefs might have bearing on health practices in relation to these health problems?
15. What are the key things people need to know to manage these problems independently, and what will I do to ensure that this knowledge is gained?

2. **Apply principles of nursing process.** For example, assess before acting, stay focused on outcomes, anticipate and change approaches as needed. Make judgments based on *fact* rather than emotions or hearsay.

3. **Develop a systematic approach to assessment.** When you're systematic, you're more efficient and less likely to overlook something. Chapter 5 will offer opportunities to practice identifying systematic approaches.

4. **Determine a system that helps you make decisions about what must be done now and what can wait until later** (see Box 3–10).
   - **Be sure you identify the underlying causes of the problems:** Until you've identified the problem *and its cause,* you don't really understand the problem or what has to be done immediately. For example, if you suspect someone's abdominal pain is caused by appendicitis, you know that a top priority in managing the situation is to consult a physician. If you treat the pain without medical evaluation, you'll mask symptoms, possibly delaying diagnosis of a serious problem
   - **Always ask yourself, Could any of these signs and symptoms be caused by a medication or problem with structure or function of an organ or system requiring medical management?** If the answer is yes, an immediate priority, before going on to plan nursing care, is to notify someone who is more knowledgeable than you are (e.g., your supervisor, an advanced practice nurse, a physician).

5. **Never perform an action if you don't know why it's indicated, why it works (the rationale), and whether there are risks of harm in the context of the current patient situation.** When you understand why an action is specified, you know whether it's relevant and appropriate. When you know risks of harm, you can identify ways of reducing the risk. For example, if you're aware of the risks of introducing an air embolism into an IV line, you find ways to reduce that risk (e.g., taping connections together).

6. **Learn from your human resources (faculty, experts, classmates, other nurses) and when in doubt, get help from a qualified professional.** Your patients' rights to expedient care take precedence over your need to learn independently. Other professionals can help you decide whether you have time to look up your concerns in a reference. You can also learn from your peers' experiences. Collaborating with classmates is a win-win situation: Asking questions like, What did you look for? How did you know what to look for? and

| BOX 3–10 | **A Common Approach to Identifying Immediate Priorities** |

Treatment for first- and second-level priorities is usually initiated in rapid succession or simultaneously. *At times,* the order of priority might change, depending on the seriousness of the problem and relationship between the problems. For example, if abnormal lab values are life-threatening, they become a higher priority; if your patient is having trouble breathing because of acute pain, managing the pain might become the highest priority. It's important to consider the *relationship* between the problems: For example, if *problem Y* causes *problem Z, problem Y* takes priority over *problem Z.*

1. **First-level priority problems** (immediate priorities): Remember the ABC'S:
   Airway problems
   Breathing problems
   Cardiac/circulation problems
   Signs (vital signs concerns)

2. **Second-level priority problems** (immediate, after treatment for first-level problems is initiated)
   Mental status change
   Acute pain
   Acute urinary elimination problems
   Untreated medical problems requiring immediate attention (e.g., a diabetic who hasn't had insulin)
   Abnormal lab values
   Risks of infection, safety, or security (for patient or for others)

Note: To help you remember the above, mnemonic MAA-U-AR provides the first letter of each of the second-level priority problems.

3. **Third-level priority problems** (later priorities)
   Health problems that don't fit into the above categories (e.g., problems with lack of knowledge, activity, rest, family coping)

What was the biggest thing you learned? will help your classmates clarify their knowledge and help you learn from being involved in real situations. **Note:** Keep in mind the ethics of discussing patient care: Don't use names or talk about patients in public places where others might overhear (e.g., cafeteria, elevators).

7. **Become familiar with facility standards (e.g., protocols, policies, procedures, critical paths) that relate to your patient's problems.**

They are intended to help you make decisions about key aspects of care.

8. **Become familiar with the technology you'll use (e.g., IV pumps, computers, monitors).** These are intended to reduce some of the work of nursing.

9. **Remember the importance of caring (being willing to place great importance on the wants and needs of patients and their significant others).** More specifically, caring has been described by patients as *vigilance* (nurse attentiveness, highly skilled practice, basic care, nurturing, and going the extra mile); *mutuality* (relationships and behaviors generated among the nurse, patient, and family); and *healing* (lifesaving behaviors and freeing the patient from anxiety and concerns).[5]

10. **Follow policies and procedures carefully with a good understanding of the reasons behind them.** These are designed to help you use good judgment.

OTHER PERSPECTIVES

Fostering Cross-Cultural Understanding

"Working successfully with a culturally diverse staff and patient population encompasses two sets of skills. First, nurses need the holistic skills to manage patients who are different from themselves. . . . However, the skill that's frequently overlooked is learning to work with diversity among staff members. Embracing cultural diversity in the workplace, as well as in the community, has to be an institutional commitment."[6]

— *Antonia Villareul, RN, PhD, FAAN*
President, National Association of Hispanic Nurses

SUMMARY

Critical thinking in nursing must be precise, disciplined thinking that promotes accuracy and depth of data collection and that seeks to clearly identify the issues at hand. To bring your understanding of this chapter together as a whole, see Table 3–2.

TABLE 3–2	**Applied Definition of Critical Thinking with Corresponding Strategies**
KEY POINTS ON CRITICAL THINKING IN NURSING	STRATEGIES
• Entails purposeful, outcome-directed (results-oriented) thinking	• Determine overall outcomes: describe exactly what will be observed in the patient, family, or group to show the benefit nursing care will make
• Is driven by patient, family, and community needs	• Decide what specific patient, family, or group needs *must* be met to achieve the overall outcomes
• Is based on principles of nursing process and scientific method	• Follow principles of assessing, diagnosing, planning, implementing, and evaluating care
• Requires specific knowledge, skills, and experience	• Apply related theoretical and experiential knowledge; consult experts and other disciplines as needed
• Is guided by professional standards and ethics codes	• Plan and give care in accordance with professional standards and ethics codes (e.g., national, local, and facility standards, practice guidelines, ethics codes)
• Requires strategies that maximize human potential and compensate for problems created by human nature	• Use client, family, and community strengths; identify ways to maximize human potential (e.g., promote independence by facilitating learning); be cognizant of how your own perspective may be influencing care (e.g., personal biases or dislikes)
• Is constantly reevaluating, self-correcting, and striving to improve	• Monitor outcomes closely, reflecting on how things could be done more efficiently

CRITICAL THINKING EXERCISES

1. Clarify how the terms *clinical judgment, clinical reasoning,* and *critical thinking* are related (5 sentences or less).*

2. Write a paragraph describing what clinical judgment entails.*

3. Give at least one reason health care delivery today is focused on customer satisfaction.*

---

*An example response for this exercise can be found in the Response Key at the back of the book beginning on page 240.

4. Figure 3–4 (page 84) provides a model to help students decide whether an act is within their scope of practice. Using this model, decide whether you're allowed to irrigate a nasogastric tube in the clinical setting.*

5. An important aspect of developing clinical judgment is being willing to recognize the importance of caring (being willing to place great importance on the wants and needs of patients and their significant others). Keeping this in mind, how would you interpret the statements made by the off-going nurse below?*

   On-coming nurse: How is the family doing?
   Off-going nurse: They seem to be fine. They're sticking to visiting hours and have been in to visit 15 minutes this morning and 15 minutes this afternoon.

6. Respond to the following from the prechapter self-test.
   a. Describe your responsibilities in relation to diagnosis and management of medical and nursing problems.*
   b. Explain the role of ethics codes and national and facility standards and guidelines in making decisions.*
   c. Identify a system to determine immediate priorities.*
   d. Develop a personal plan to help you develop sound clinical judgment.*

   *An example response for this exercise can be found in the Response Key at the back of the book beginning on page 240.

KEY POINTS

- Key points of the applied definition of critical thinking can be found on page 58.

- While problem-solving skills are required for critical thinking, to succeed in today's competitive workplace, you can't be satisfied with just having a "problem-solving mentality." You also need a sincere desire to improve.

- Critical thinking in nursing constantly strives to improve by focusing on two key questions: (1) What are the outcomes? and (2) How could we achieve these outcomes more efficiently?

- Because the conclusions and decisions we as nurses make *affect people's lives*, our thinking must be guided by sound reasoning—precise, disciplined thinking that promotes accuracy and depth of data collection and that seeks to clearly identify the issues at hand.

- Understanding how novice thinking differs from expert thinking helps us set realistic goals for developing critical thinking ability.

- Care delivery has moved from a *diagnose and treat (DT)* to a *predict, prevent, and manage (PPM)* that focuses on prevention through identification of risk factors and *early* intervention.

- Care today is focused on outcomes and based on evidence. We must be able to answer questions like, (1) Exactly what are the expected outcomes? (2) By when do you expect to achieve these outcomes? and (3) What evidence is there that indicates you're likely to achieve these outcomes?

- Experts use the nursing process in a very dynamic way because they know what steps can be safely skipped or delayed. They also know when situations warrant a rigorous, comprehensive, step-by-step approach.

- You *must* be familiar with principles of nursing process and care planning to be able to know whether the plan of care is sufficiently documented.

- Care plans include four major components: (1) major outcomes of nursing care, (2) actual and potential problems, (3) specific interventions, and (4) evaluation or progress notes.

- We have moved from "nurses diagnose and treat only nursing diagnoses" to "nurses diagnose and manage various problems, depending on their knowledge, expertise, and qualifications."

- The terms *diagnose* and *diagnosis* have legal implications. They imply that there's a spe-cific problem that requires management by a qualified expert (see rule, page 74).

- Understanding *conceptually* the types of problems that nurses focus on is an important step toward understanding your responsibilities related to diagnosis and management of health problems. Page 75 lists examples of the types of problems that nurses commonly manage.

- Some schools and facilities have made significant improvements in identifying nursing problems by using NANDA-recommended nursing diagnostic labels, while others focus more on nursing responsibilities in the context of medical problems and use of critical paths.

- As you study (or work in) different specialty practices, for example, maternity nursing, you need to check with experts, up-to-date texts, and policies and procedures to determine the types of problems you're expected to diagnose and manage.

- To be sure you detect both nursing and possible medical problems use both a nursing model and a body systems approach to collecting data (see Boxes 3–5 and 3–6 and Fig. 3–3).

- The terms *clinical judgment, clinical reasoning,* and *critical thinking* are often used interchangeably. Actually you *use* clinical reasoning and critical thinking to make a clinical judgment.

- *Clinical judgment* has two meanings: (1) **nursing opinion(s)** made about a person's, family's, or group's health at a certain point in time and (2) **nursing decisions** made about things like what to assess, what health data suggest, what to do first, and who should do it.

- Ability to make clinical judgments depends on theoretical and experiential knowledge— for example, knowing what to look for, how to recognize when a patient's status is changing, and what to do about it.

- Clinical judgment includes knowing when the situation requires more than "thinking on your feet" (e.g., knowing when you need to take more time or get additional opinions).

- Developing clinical reasoning skills takes time. It also requires a commitment to study common health problems, seek out clinical experiences, and come prepared to the clinical setting.

 CRITICAL MOMENT

Connect with people by letting them know your human side and imagining what it would be like to be in their shoes.

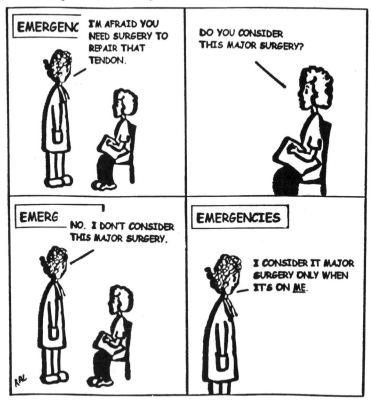

© R. Alfaro-LeFevre 1998.

Footnotes

[1]Jenks, J. (1998, August). Verbal communication.

[2]Norman, G. (1988). Problem-solving skills, solving problems and problem-based learning. *Medical Education, 22,* 280.

[3]North American Nursing Diagnosis Association. (1997). *Nursing diagnosis: Definitions and classifications.* Philadelphia: Author, p. 4.

[4]Nash, D. (1998). Email communication. July.

[5]Burfitt, S., Greiner, D., and Miers, L. (1993). Professional nurse caring as perceived by critically ill patients: A phenomenologic study. *American Journal of Critical Care, 2*(6), 489–499.

[6]Campion, C. (1998). Embracing our differences. *Nursing Spectrum FL Ed., 8*(14), 5.

See comprehensive bibliography beginning on page 280.

4

Critical Thinking in Nursing: Beyond Clinical Judgment

This chapter at a glance . . .

Read the Learning Outcomes listed below and decide whether you can readily achieve each one. If you can, you don't need to read this chapter and can go on to Chapter 5. Don't be concerned if you can't achieve any of the objectives at this time. We'll come back to these outcomes later in the chapter, in Critical Thinking Exercises.

LEARNING OUTCOMES

After completing this chapter, you should be able to:

- Give a description and an example of the terms *moral uncertainty, moral dilemma*, and *moral distress*.
- Make prudent decisions based on ethical principles, codes, and practice standards.
- Describe your responsibilities in relation to nursing research.
- Explain why it's important to choose refereed or peer-reviewed journals when looking for research articles.
- Explain how to decide whether you know enough to apply research findings to practice.
- Use critical thinking to create a teaching plan.
- Address the roles of memorizing and reasoning in teaching ourselves.
- Describe five strategies that can help you improve your test scores.

ABSTRACT

This chapter continues the discussion of critical thinking in nursing begun in Chapter 3. It begins by addressing how changes in health care have heightened the awareness of the need for moral and ethical reasoning skills. It then goes on to address how to apply research to practice and give strategies for teaching others, teaching ourselves, and test taking.

Having defined critical thinking in nursing and examined how to develop clinical judgment, let's go on to examine reasoning in the five other common nursing situations.

- Moral and ethical reasoning
- Nursing research
- Teaching others
- Teaching ourselves
- Test taking

Let's begin with moral and ethical reasoning.

MORAL AND ETHICAL REASONING

As health care becomes more complex, we are more aware that nurses often find themselves in situations where they need to have sound moral and ethical reasoning skills. Think about the Other Perspectives that follow:

OTHER PERSPECTIVES

Ethical Challenges Facing Nurses

"In an era of health care reform, rapid scientific and technologic advances, a growing aging population, limited resources and preeminence (dominance) of patient autonomy, nurses are confronted with many challenges.

"Questions related to the right to refuse treatment, advance directives, the use of artificially provided nutrition and hydration, participation in research protocols, genetic advances, allocation of scarce resources and quality of life are commonplace. Today, with the array of choices available, nurses are called upon to be actively involved with the patient and family in the decision-making process.

"Nurses grapple daily with a maze of ethical uncertainties and quandaries associated with the delivery of health care. To deal with the ethical ramifications of practice, nurses must be adequately prepared. . . . As the most omnipresent health care provider, the nurse is often the first to become aware of many ethical predicaments. Nurses confront conflicting loyalties, unanswered questions and ethical ambiguities."[1]   —*Colleen Scanlon, JD, MS, RN*

"Nurses are often at the intersection where patients, families, and other health care professionals struggle with decisions about medical treatments and appropriate use of patient care technologies.

"The consequences of such decisions are significant for patients, for their families and loved ones, for nurses and other care providers and for the delivery of health services. . . . Ethical questions may involve conflicts of values, obligations, loyalties, interests, or needs in a patient care situation such as disagreement between health team members, patient, family or loved ones about the use of aggressive and costly therapies."[2]

—*Mila Ann Aroskar, EdD, RN, FAAN*

As evident from the above quotes, these are challenging times that require a solid understanding of what's involved in making moral and ethical decisions.

Moral versus Ethical Reasoning

Moral reasoning and *ethical reasoning* are often used interchangeably. However, there is a slight difference between these two terms. Think about the difference in the following ways these two terms are described:

- **Moral reasoning:** Refers to judgments made based on *personal* standards of right and wrong (e.g., I personally believe it's okay to tell little white lies now and then).
- **Ethical reasoning:** Refers to judgments made by applying standards derived from the formal study of what criteria ought to be used to determine whether actions are justified and therefore morally right or wrong (e.g., I personally don't think that there's anything wrong with little white lies now and then, but most ethicists will tell you it's wrong to lie to patients).

Here's another example:

Case Scenario

Suppose you're admitting a young woman who is freely and knowledgeably seeking a tubal ligation. Morally (according to your personal standards), you feel sterilization is wrong. However, as a nurse, you realize that ethically this woman has a right to make this choice and that it would be inappropriate for you to tell her sterilization is wrong or for you to try to get her to change her mind.

How Do You Decide?

So how *do* you make decisions about moral and ethical issues? The answer is, *with great difficulty.* Okay, so I'm only kidding, but sometimes thinking about these types of issues is so stressful that we could use a little humor. Let's get serious and look at what you do when you're faced with situations that have no easily agreed upon *right* answers. Rather, each answer has its own merits and weaknesses, and it's difficult to say that one is really better than another.

Moral and ethical problems may be divided into three categories[3]:

- **Moral uncertainty:** You aren't sure which moral principles or values apply. *Example:* A patient asks you whether you think his doctor is a good doctor. You don't think the doctor is very competent. Do you tell him?
- **Moral dilemma:** You're faced with a situation in which you have two (or more) choices available, but neither (or none) of them seems satisfactory. *Example:* A doctor tells *you* she's sure your friend has cancer but tells *your friend,* "I won't know anything until the diagnosis is made by the lab, next week." When your friend begs you to tell him what the doctor knows, what do you do? If you tell him you don't know, you're lying. If you tell him what the doctor told you, you risk breaking his trust in his physician.
- **Moral distress:** You know the right thing to do, but institutional constraints make it nearly impossible to do what is right. *Example:* You know a patient isn't ready for discharge and that his wife is hopelessly unprepared to care for him. When you report this problem to the physician, you're told the hospital has "no choice" but to discharge him. What do you do?

So, did you know what you'd do in the above examples? If so, on what did you base your decisions? Gut feelings? Personal values and standards? Professional standards?

Making moral and ethical decisions requires knowledge of ethics codes and principles. You can't be impulsive or act on the basis of feelings. As a nurse, you must clearly understand standards and principles that guide moral and ethical decision making. You must be able to justify your actions to others by ethical argumentation.

Principles and Standards for Making Ethical Decisions

Like in *Snow White,* there are seven "dwarfs" (seven commonly cited principles, actually) that guide ethical decision making: autonomy, beneficence, justice, fidelity, veracity, confidentiality, and accountability. Here's a description of each one.

- **Autonomy.** The belief that people have the right to be self-determining and to make legally acceptable decisions based on:
  - their *own* values and beliefs
  - adequate information that is given free from coercion
  - sound reasoning that considers all the alternatives
- **Beneficence.** The intent of benefiting others and avoiding harm.
- **Justice.** The intent of treating all people fairly and giving what is due or owed.
- **Fidelity.** The importance of keeping promises and not making promises you can't keep.
- **Veracity (Truth Telling).** The importance of honesty and truth telling.
- **Confidentiality.** Respecting the privacy of information.
- **Accountability.** Being willing to be accountable for the consequences of your actions.

Standards, Ethics Codes, Bills of Rights, Advance Directives

In addition to the above principles, standards, ethics codes, and bills of rights guide ethical conduct. For example, the American Nurses Association's *Standards of Nursing Practice* (Standard V) states[4]:

"The nurse:
- "Is guided by *Code for Nurses**
- "Maintains client confidentiality; acts as client advocate; delivers care in a nonjudgmental and nondiscriminatory manner that's sensitive to client diversity; preserves/protects client autonomy,

---

*See page 268 (Appendix F) for American Nurses Association Code for Nurses.

dignity, and rights; seeks resources to help formulate ethical decisions."

Ethically, you're required to maintain acceptable standards of practice. By taking the nursing role, you must see that your patients and clients receive competent care. Therefore, standards addressing how care should be given in specific situations (policies, procedures, and specialty practice standards) play an important part in delivering ethical care.

Bills of rights such as the American Hospital Association's *A Patient's Bill of Rights* (see pages 268 to 271) and other bills of rights[5] (e.g., Pregnant Patient's Bill of Rights, Indian Patient's Bill of Rights, a Nursing Home Bill of Rights, and Veteran's Administration Code of Patient Concern) also act as guides for how you respond to ethical issues.

Advance Directives (see Box 4–1) help us make decisions about cardiac resuscitation and other end-of-life treatments as noted in the Critical Moments that follow.

CRITICAL MOMENTS

Advance Directives Promote Patient Autonomy

Too many people wait until it's too late to address advance directives. Think and talk about it now with your loved ones. Doing so helps ensure that your wishes are followed if you're ever in a situation where those making decisions for you find it hard to refuse aggressive treatment that merely prolongs your dying. It will also help you have peace of mind if you're ever asked to choose among treatment options for your loved ones.

BOX 4–1	**What Are Advance Directives?**

Advance directives include two documents*:

Living Will: Designates the types of medical treatments you would or wouldn't want in specific instances (for example, whether you want to continue ventilator support if you become permanently unconscious).

Durable Power of Attorney for Health Care (DPAHC): Identifies who you want to make treatment decisions if there comes a time when you aren't able to do so.

*These two documents may be combined into one document, called the *combination directive.*

You now have an idea of the principles and standards that guide moral and ethical decision making. Let's go on to some steps that can help you develop a comprehensive, thoughtful approach to moral and ethical reasoning.

Steps for Moral and Ethical Reasoning

1. **Clearly identify the problem or issue based on the perspectives of the key players involved.** For example, Mrs. Pizzi, an elderly woman who lives alone, tells you she doesn't want her leg amputated and that she'd rather die than live as an amputee. Her daughter tells you her mother is incompetent to make this decision. *Problem:* Who has the right to make this decision? Is Mrs. Pizzi competent? Does she have the right to refuse surgery? Does the daughter have the right to overrule her mother?

2. **Decide what your role will be.** For example, is an ethical board involved? Does this family rely heavily on your judgment? Do you just need to listen?

3. **Recognize your personal values and how they may influence your ability to participate in health care decision making.** For example, in Mrs. Pizzi's case, do you believe no one has the right to refuse lifesaving surgery? If so, how would this affect your ability to help Mrs. Pizzi with this decision? If you can't be objective, let your supervisor know so that another caregiver can assist with decision making.

4. **Identify the alternatives.** For example, is it possible to delay this decision? Would Mrs. Pizzi be willing to have the surgery if the daughter commits to caring for her? Would more time spent with the daughter help her to understand and support her mother's wishes? Could social services help? Should we request an ethics consult?

5. **Determine the outcomes (consequences) of the alternatives.** For example, if the decision is delayed, will it be detrimental to health? Would the daughter indeed be able to care for her mother?

6. **List the alternatives and rate them according to which would produce the least harm or greatest good, based on client and family values.** To do so, don't consider good versus bad. Instead, ask where each fits on the following scale:

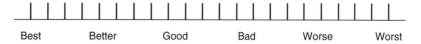

| Best | Better | Good | Bad | Worse | Worst |

The above scale will help you distinguish between choices that at first glance might seem equally moral.

7. **Develop a plan of action that will facilitate the best choices.** In situations where the choices are all good, choose the one that is the *greater good.* In situations where none of the choices are really good, choose the one that is the *lesser evil.*

8. **Put the plan into action and monitor the response closely.**

To complete this section on moral and ethical reasoning, study Box 4–2, which answers key critical thinking questions in relation to moral and ethical decision making.

CRITICAL MOMENT

Breech of Privacy May Cause Legal Problems

We know that ethically, nurses are bound to keep patient information private. Patient privacy is also a *legal* concern. If you divulge private information, you could find yourself involved in a lawsuit. Carefully guard patients' rights to privacy.

■ **Want to Know More?** Here are some resources you can contact to learn more about how to get help, publications, and educational programs on moral and ethical reasoning:

ANA Center for Ethics and Human Rights
600 Maryland Ave. SW, Suite 100 West
Washington, DC 20024
202-651-7055

National Reference Center for Bioethics Literature
Kennedy Institute of Ethics
Georgetown University
Washington, DC 20057
800-MED-ETHX
Internet: http://guweb.georgetown.edu/nrcbl

The Hastings Center
Route 9D
Garrison, NY 10524-5555
914-424-4040

| BOX 4–2 | **Moral and Ethical Reasoning: Key Questions*** |

1. **What major outcomes (observable results) do I/we expect to see in this particular person, family, or group?** The patient (or person designated to make treatment decisions) will be able to express that he has made an informed, uncoerced, well-reasoned, legally acceptable decision based on his values and believed to promote his interests.

2. **What problems or issues *must* be addressed to achieve the major outcomes?** *What's* the main issue (be sure to understand *when*, *where*, and *how* the issue developed)? How can we be sure the key players are well informed, have considered all the alternatives, and understand the short- and long-range consequences of each alternative?

3. **What are the circumstances?** *Who* are the key players (e.g., patient, family, caregivers, payors)? *What* is your role (facility policies and procedures are likely to affect your role)? *What* are the morally significant variables present (e.g., beliefs, values, and preferences of the participants; cultural, religious, and economic considerations; interests of all involved parties)?

4. **What knowledge is required?** Required knowledge includes:
   - Ethical theory and related principles, standards of care, professional codes of ethics (e.g., ANA and CNA codes of ethics, Patient's Bill of Rights, etc.)
   - Ethical decision-making framework (see page 105)
   - Communication skills

5. **How much room is there for error?** Room for error *varies* according to the consequences of the decision. For example, in which situation below do you think you have more room for error?
   a. You're deliberating about a patient's capacity to make an informed, voluntary decision about stopping life-sustaining therapies.
   b. You're deliberating about a patient's capacity to make an informed, voluntary decision about choosing among chemotherapies with different probabilities of success and side effects.

   If you thought *b*, you're correct. In situation *a*, you're deciding whether the person has the capacity to decide whether to live or die, leaving little room for error. In situation *b*, you're deciding whether the person has the capacity to choose among therapy options, some of which may be better matched to his values and interests.

6. **How much time do I have?** Time frame for decision making is also a factor of the consequences of the decision at hand. For example, if the parents of a sick child withhold consent for treatment, there's more time to deliberate if the child's life isn't in immediate jeopardy.

*Answers to questions provided by Carol Taylor, PhD, MSN, Healthcare Ethicist and Assistant Professor, Nursing, Georgetown University, Washington, DC. *Box continued on following page*

BOX 4–2	**Moral and Ethical Reasoning: Key Questions** *Continued*

7. **What resources can help me?** Human resources include clinical ethicists, ethics committees, clinical nurse educators, nursing faculty, facility policies on ethics, and librarians. Other resources include articles, ethics texts, computer data bases, and organizations that promote the study of ethics (see *Want to know more?*, page 106).

8. **Whose perspectives must be considered?** The most significant perspective to consider is that of the patient. Other important perspectives include the family and significant others, caregivers, relevant third parties (e.g., insurers), and professional groups who have addressed the issues (e.g., those who have developed professional ethics codes as above and the Hastings Center).

9. **What's influencing my thinking?** Thinking may be influenced by conscious or unconscious bias, discrimination, personal motives, or fear of legal liability (e.g., I've got to restrain this person or he may fall, and I'll be sued). Thinking may also be influenced by any of the factors listed in Table 2–1, Factors Influencing Critical Thinking Ability (page 30).

NURSING RESEARCH

Based as much as possible on strict rules of the scientific method, research is one of the most rigorous and disciplined uses of critical thinking in nursing. Researchers must have a variety of highly developed critical thinking skills, from knowing how to clearly identify the problem or issue to be studied to determining the best way to collect meaningful data, to analyzing and interpreting the data. Think about the following definition:

What is research?

Research is diligent, systematic inquiry or investigation to validate and refine existing knowledge and generate new knowledge. The concepts *systematic* and *diligent* are critical to the meaning of research because they imply planning, organization, and persistence.[6]

As in many professions, nursing research is accomplished by a comparatively small group of dedicated, highly qualified nurses who are willing to commit themselves to a lengthy, sometimes costly process.

So, you might wonder, If research is conducted by a relatively small group of expert nurses, how important is it for beginning nurses? The answer is, *very important*. Research is essential to advancing nursing practice. It helps us generate a body of knowledge that provides a scientific basis for planning, predicting, and controlling the outcomes of nursing practice.[7] Its importance is emphasized by the inclusion of *using research* as a standard of performance set forth by the American Nurses Association (ANA) (see Standard VII, Appendix F, page 267). By listing research as a *standard of performance*, the ANA sends the message that all nurses are expected to use research findings whenever appropriate.

Although it's beyond the scope of this chapter to address how to actually *conduct* research studies, this section focuses on how to *use* research findings. Let's begin by addressing the questions, What is the role of beginning nurses in relation to research? and How do you decide whether you can safely use research findings?

Questions and Answers on Beginning Nurses' Research Role

1. **What is the role of beginning nurses in relation to nursing research?** Beginning nurses have four main responsibilities:
   - **To think analytically about the situations they encounter and seek out research results that might improve nursing care.** For example, if you frequently care for people with postoperative leg edema after heart bypass surgery, you might think, I wonder if there are any research studies explaining why this happens and what can be done about it? To answer this question, you might simply be able to consult your instructor, a clinical nurse educator, or nurse researcher. Even if you don't have time to go to the library, often these people will help you.
   - **To raise questions about their practice that might prompt a researcher to formulate a question to guide a study.** For example, you could ask your supervisor, Since we seem to be having an increase in infections, would it be worthwhile to study whether our procedure for hand washing is really effective?
   - **To help researchers collect data.** If you're asked to record certain information in the clinical area, it's your professional responsibility to do so, diligently and accurately, as long as it doesn't interfere with nursing care.
   - **To continue to acquire and share knowledge related to research.** We must constantly be asking ourselves questions like, Am I mak-

ing time to become familiar with research related to the clinical situations in which I'm involved? and Do I interact with others (peers, educators) to learn more about research? For those of you who find reading research articles tedious, get started by talking with peers and educators or perhaps joining a journal club. This helps you to learn in a dynamic, stimulating environment. Once you learn the basics, meeting your responsibilities in relation to research becomes easier, more interesting, and even an enjoyable challenge!

2. **If I have limited knowledge of research, how do I know whether there are research studies I should be using in my practice?** The following will help you answer this question.

   • **Recognize that research findings must not be used indiscriminately.** Before you can use research results, you must decide whether the study is valid and reliable (whether it was conducted in such a way that you can trust that the results are accurate). For example, how often have you heard a commercial that proclaims, "In a recent research study, our product was proven to be more effective than the other leading products." Do you believe every one of these commercials? Probably not. As independent thinkers, you must always ask questions to determine whether you can apply the results of *any* research study.

   • **Search the literature for research articles related to your area of practice.** The first time you do this, take a partner with you to the library and tackle the search collaboratively.

   • **Choose refereed or peer-reviewed journals (journals that publish articles only after they've been reviewed by experts).** This usually can be found in the front of the journal where you find information like who is on the editorial board, who is the publisher, and so on. These journals are more likely to have reliable information.

   • **Scan first to eliminate irrelevant articles; then read the ones that seem as though they'd be most useful.** Learning how to scan then read research articles efficiently helps you avoid becoming overwhelmed trying to do too much at one time. To learn how to choose relevant research articles more easily and how to decide whether you know enough to use a specific study's results, review Boxes 4–3 and 4–4.

Box 4–5 gives strategies for increasing research utilization in practice.

BOX 4–3	**How to Scan, Then Read Research Articles**

Scanning to find useful research articles saves time by helping you eliminate irrelevant articles without having to read them in their entirety.

1. **Read the abstract first: This summarizes the issues, methods, and results.** If the abstract isn't applicable to your clinical problem, you might choose to read no further.
2. **If the abstract seems applicable, skip to the end of the article;** then scan the article by reading the information under the following headings in the order listed below:
   a. Summary (may also be listed as Conclusions)
   b. Discussion
   c. Nursing Implications
   d. Suggestions For Further Research
   You may be able to eliminate articles just by reading any of the above headings.
3. **If the information you've scanned is relevant, go on to read the entire study.** Give yourself plenty of time and don't be discouraged if you find sections you don't understand. Instead, take notes on what you *do* understand. Come back to the more difficult sections at another time, after getting help from an expert or textbook (or both).

BOX 4–4	**Questions to Ask Yourself to Decide Whether You Know Enough about a Research Article to Use the Results**

1. **Have I checked whether the article comes from a journal that's peer or expert reviewed?**
2. **Do I understand:**
   - What's already known about the topic
   - What the researchers studied and why and how they studied it
   - What they found out and whether the results are valid
   - What the results imply and how they apply to my particular clinical situation
3. **Do I know how the results of this study compare with the results of other, similar studies?** If other studies produced similar findings, the probability that the results are *reliable* increases.

BOX 4–5	**Strategies for Getting Research into Practice***

- Identify common areas of need in the clinical setting.
- Review research studies that provide knowledge about the identified areas.
- Provide education and reviews for nurses on how to read, critique, and understand clinical implications of research.
- Determine relevance of research to setting and patient type.
- Devise protocols for placing knowledge into practice and defining expected outcomes.
- Provide education needed to place protocols into practice.
- Evaluate and adjust practice protocol.
- Identify areas in need of further investigation.

*Data from Goode, C., Lovett, M., Hayes, J., Butcher, L. (1997). Use of research based knowledge in clinical practice. *Journal of Nursing Administration, 17*(12), 11–17.

Quality Improvement

Quality improvement (QI), a responsibility of all nurses, is perhaps the type of research most frequently encountered in the clinical setting. Most facilities have a department that is responsible for ongoing studies designed to improve outcomes. For example, through quality improvement studies, some nurses have shown that delays in medications coming from pharmacy may significantly increase lengths of hospital stays. As a result policies and procedures have changed to ensure that medications come to the units in a timely fashion, and lengths of stays have decreased.

QI studies usually study information from three different perspectives:

1. **Outcome evaluation (focuses on results).** For example, asking, How many of our patients undergoing bowel surgery experienced an infection that was serious enough to delay discharge?
2. **Process evaluation (focuses on how care was given).** For example, asking, At what point were our patients undergoing bowel surgery first given antibiotics?
3. **Structure evaluation (focuses on setting).** For example, asking, In what setting were antibiotics first given (emergency department? operating room? surgical unit?)?

Your responsibilities in relation to QI are the same as the previously listed responsibilities for research.

To complete this section, review Box 4–6, which answers key critical thinking questions in relation to using nursing research.

BOX 4–6	**Using Nursing Research: Key Questions**

1. **What major outcomes (observable results) do I/we plan to achieve?** After studying available nursing research, I/we will be able to improve nursing practices or understand more about a nursing concern.

2. **What problems or issues *must* be addressed to achieve the major outcomes?** Example problems or issues include, How can we find the best practice and research articles for this particular information? How can we make time to do the work involved? Are there policies and procedures on putting research into practice we must follow? What are the risks of applying this research to our practice? How can we ensure that we proceed safely?

3. **What are the circumstances?** For example, how urgent is the problem? In what setting are you planning to use the research findings? What are the characteristics of your patient population (age, sex, etc.)?

4. **What knowledge is required?** Required knowledge includes whether the research article comes from a refereed or peer-reviewed journal, familiarity with the topic, previous research on the topic, research methods, and (for some research designs) statistical analysis. You also need to be familiar with the following library resources: indexes, catalogs, computer search services, interlibrary loan services, circulation department, reference department, and audiovisual services.

5. **How much room is there for error?** Room for error depends on how you plan to use the research results. For example, in which of the following situations do you think you have more room for error?

   a. You're reviewing available research to determine what colors have a calming effect so that hospitals can choose calming colors for their walls.

   b. You're reviewing available research to determine the best ways to prevent postoperative breathing complications so that you can include these methods in facility guidelines for postoperative care.

   If you thought *a*, you're correct. Little harm can occur if you're incorrect about the best colors, but if you're incorrect about how to best manage postoperative breathing complications, lives may be in jeopardy.

6. **How much time do I have?** The time frame depends on deadlines. Be careful to be realistic. Reviewing and analyzing research studies for application to practice is time consuming.

7. **What resources can help me?** Human resources include nurse researchers, clinical nurse educators, clinical nurse specialists, faculty, preceptors, peers, journal clubs, and librarians. Other resources are research texts, journal articles, and computer data bases.

8. **Whose perspectives must be considered?** You need to carefully consider patient, nursing, and financial perspectives of using the research.

9. **What's influencing my thinking?** Thinking may be influenced by a vested interest in the results or by a feeling of being too overwhelmed with other nursing duties to devote time to applying research. It may also be influenced by any of the factors listed in Table 2–1, Factors Influencing Critical Thinking Ability (page 30).

OTHER PERSPECTIVES

Improving Care for the Terminally Ill

"[At our facility] we decided our role is to be a patient advocate and to be able to help patients have what they think is most important in the dying process. . . . [When patients are terminal] vital signs are measured only once a day. Daily weights aren't done and blood for tests isn't routinely drawn. IV's aren't restarted unless needed for pain relief medication. Patients aren't routinely turned except when it will ease pain."[8]

–K. Janssen, RN
Case Manager and Quality Improvement Nurse

CRITICAL THINKING EXERCISES

Moral and Ethical Reasoning Exercises

1. Decide what you'd do if you had been "Me" in the following scenario*:

> **Case Scenario**
>
> My father was admitted to an intensive care unit. They didn't expect him to live. I was approached by the physician, who said, "Do you want us to resuscitate him if he arrests again?" Since my father never wanted to talk about these things, I didn't know what he'd want. I also didn't feel it was my place to answer. I called my mother and asked her the question. Here's how the conversation went.
>
> **Me:** Mom, they want to know if they should resuscitate Dad if he arrests again.
> **Mom:** You don't know what you're asking me.
> **Me:** Yes, I do. I know it's hard, but you're supposed to speak *in his voice.* Not what you want–what you think *he* wants.
> **Mom:** That's the problem. You see, all my life when I've tried to guess his decisions, he's always done just the opposite. Even when I've said to myself, "I think he'll do (whatever) only because it's the opposite of what I think he'd do," I've still been wrong.

---

*An example response for this exercise can be found in the Response Key at the back of the book beginning on page 241.

2. Which of the seven moral and ethical principles (autonomy, benefi-cence, justice, fidelity, veracity, confidentiality, accountability) apply to the following statement? (More than one may apply.)*

   By choosing the role of a nurse, you must see that your patients and clients receive competent care.

3. Respond to the following from the prechapter self-test.
   a. Describe what moral uncertainty, moral dilemma, and moral dis-tress mean and give your own example of each.

   b. Make a prudent decision based on ethical principles, codes, and practice. To achieve this outcome, together with a partner or in a group, consider the following situation:

   > **Case Scenario**
   >
   > The Blancos have cared for their 40-year-old daughter, Marilou, at home for 20 years, since she became totally comatose after a car accident. All diagnostic stud-ies indicate that Marilou will never regain consciousness. The Blancos are almost 80 years old. Because they are concerned that they won't be able to care for her, they are considering stopping tube feedings and allowing her to die. Because the family has relied heavily on your decisions for the past five years, they ask you what to do. Decide how you can best help the Blancos make this decision.

Nursing Research Exercises
1. Acquaint yourself with "big picture" research reviews. Scan the sec-tion called *Research for Practice* in recent issues of the *American Jour-nal of Nursing*. Choose one that you find interesting. Then:
   a. Summarize in your own words what the researchers studied, what they found, how it *might* be used in practice, and what questions are raised by the summary.

   b. Determine where you can find out more about the research topic, so that you can apply the study to practice.*

---

*An example response for this exercise can be found in the Response Key at the back of the book beginning on page 241.

2. Analyze a research article to apply the findings to practice. Find an article that sounds interesting. Decide:
   a. Whether you can safely apply the findings to practice.

   b. Where you can find more information on the topic.

   c. What questions reading the article raises.

3. Respond to the following from the prechapter self-test.
   a. Describe your responsibilities in relation to nursing research.
   b. Explain why it's important to choose refereed or peer-reviewed journals when looking for research articles.*
   c. Explain how to decide whether you know enough to apply research findings to practice.

---

*An example response for this exercise can be found in the Response Key at the back of the book beginning on page 241.

TEACHING OTHERS

Creative critical thinking is essential to teaching people the information they need to be independent. People today are discharged sicker and quicker than they were in the past, and many receive health care on an outpatient basis. Our teaching must be timely and effective. We must be able to clearly identify what *must* be learned and then initiate a plan that draws on client strengths.

The following steps can help you think critically about how to teach others:

1. **Be clear about the desired outcome: what exactly will the person be able to do when you complete your teaching?** The person will be able to regulate insulin dosage based on blood glucose readings.
2. **Decide (1) *what* exactly the person must learn to achieve the desired outcome and (2) what the best way is for him to learn it.**
   * Clarify *with the person* what is already known.
   * Determine readiness to learn: Ask what their biggest concerns are and *listen carefully.*

- Determine preferred learning styles (e.g., doing, observing, listening, or reading) and use this information to plan teaching. For example, if you're teaching injection technique and they're doers, have them start by *doing* something, like handling a syringe. If they'd rather read, start by giving them a pamphlet.
- Identify barriers to learning (e.g., consider language, reading skills, developmental problems, or problems with motivation).
- Encourage them to ask questions, get involved, and let you know how they'd like to learn. For example, you could say, Let me know if you have a better way of learning this. Not everyone learns the same way.

3. **Reduce anxiety by offering support.** An example is saying something like, Everyone is nervous when first learning to change dressings, but once you've done it a couple of times, it will be much easier.
4. **Minimize distractions and teach at appropriate times.** For example, pick a quiet room and choose times when the learners are likely to be comfortable and rested.
5. **Use pictures, diagrams, and illustrations.** These visual aids enhance comprehension and are better remembered.
6. **Create mental images by using analogies and metaphors.** For example, Insulin is like a key that opens the cell's door to allow sugar to enter. If you don't have the key (insulin), the sugar can't get into the cell. The cell starves, and sugar accumulates in the blood.
7. **Encourage people to remember by using whatever words best trigger their mind.** For example, someone might say, I need to have three things: the *soaking-dressing stuff*, the *scrubbing stuff*, and the *after-dressing stuff*.
8. **Keep it simple.** The explain-it-to-me-as-if-I-were-a-four-year-old approach works especially well for complex situations. If you can't make it simple, you're not ready to teach it.
9. **Tune into your learners' responses and change the pace, techniques, or content if needed.** For example, if they've forgotten important content, take time to review it; if they don't seem to understand what you're saying, write it down or draw a picture.
10. **Summarize key points and don't leave learners empty-handed.** Even the best learners may have trouble remembering what they've just been taught. Give them the important points in writing so they can refresh their memory later.

To complete this section, review Box 4–7, which answers key critical thinking questions in relation to teaching others.

BOX 4–7	**Teaching Others: Key Questions**

1. **What major outcomes(observable results)do I/we plan to achieve?** After I/we finish teaching, and with the help of notes if necessary, the person (or caregiver) will be able to demonstrate mastery of the required information or skill.
2. **What problems or issues *must* be addressed to achieve the major outcomes?** What exactly must be learned? Is the person ready to learn or are there other issues to be dealt with, such as anger, denial, or anxiety? What's this person's (or caregiver's) motivation (does he or she understand why it is necessary to learn the information or skill)? What's this person's (or caregiver's) preferred learning style? Are there other barriers to learning, for example, language or literacy barriers?
3. **What are the circumstances?** *Who* must you teach (adult, child, elderly person)? How complex is the information to be learned? Are you dealing with real or simulated situations? Does the person have previous experiences related to what must be learned?
4. **What knowledge is required?** Required knowledge includes familiarity with content to be taught, communication skills, and teaching and learning principles.
5. **How much room is there for error?** Room for error *varies* according to the consequences of what happens if the learner doesn't master the information. For example, in which situation below do you think you have more room for error?
   a. You're teaching insulin injection technique to someone who's basically healthy and whose daughter is an ICU nurse who's willing to monitor injection technique at home.
   b. You're teaching insulin injection technique to someone who has a compromised immune system and lives alone with no relatives.

   If you thought *a,* you're correct. If the person in situation *b* goes home without mastering insulin technique, he may not manage his diabetes, and he may also develop an infection. Therefore, you must be *sure* his injection technique is meticulous.

OTHER PERSPECTIVES

Teaching "Why" Promotes Independence

"[People] need to know why the things we ask them to do are important; then they can figure out how they can incorporate them into their daily life. [For example] understanding why the insulin dose must be balanced with food and activity allows them the ability to make decisions about how they will do it. It's their disease. Orders won't work. They must be empowered with the ability to think and problem-solve for themselves."[9]

—*Paula Cot Yutzy, RN*

BOX 4–7	**Teaching Others: Key Questions *Continued***

6. **How much time do I have?** The time frame for teaching depends on when the patient will be discharged from care. For example, if by day 3 the person is expected to be discharged, you have 3 days to teach the required information, or home care visits will be required.

7. **What resources can help me?** Human resources include clinical nurse educators, clinical nurse specialists, preceptors, more experienced nurses, peers, librarians, and other health care professionals (pharmacists, nutritionists, physical therapists, physicians). The learners are also valuable resources (it's not unusual for them to be the ones who can best identify what must be learned and how they can best learn it). Other resources include texts, articles, computerized learning packages, pamphlets, audiovisuals, and facility documents (e.g., teaching guidelines, standards of care).

8. **Whose perspectives must be considered?** The most significant perspective to consider is that of the learners: What is it they think they need to learn? How do they learn best? What are motivating factors for them to learn (e.g., some people need a deadline or a test)? Another perspective to consider is your own (e.g., how *you* feel you can best teach the material).

9. **What's influencing my thinking?** A major influencing factor is whether the learners think they can learn and whether *you* think you can be successful in helping them (both can be self-fulfilling prophecies). Thinking may also be influenced by any of the factors listed in Table 2–1, Factors Influencing Critical Thinking Ability (page 30).

Lay Terms Get the Message Across
"My sister, a mother of three children, consulted with a podiatrist about the pain she was experiencing in her toe. As the physician examined her foot, he asked, 'Which toe hurts?' Not knowing the medical terminology to answer his question, she blurted out, 'The one who went to market.'"[10]
—*Cathy Snyder, RN, BSN*

TEACHING OURSELVES

Today's challenging workplace requires that we know how to teach ourselves. We must be able to identify what it is we must learn and then find ways to learn it efficiently.

Using critical thinking when we learn, or reasoning our way through the learning process, helps us connect with our own unique way of making information *ours*. Think about the following description.

 OTHER PERSPECTIVES

Using Reasoning to Learn

Richard Paul describes using reasoning to learn as going something like this: "Let's see, how can I understand this? Is it to be understood on the model of this experience or that? Shall I think of it in this way or that? Let me see. Ah, I think I see. It's just so . . . but, no, not exactly. Let me try again. Perhaps I can understand it from this point of view, by interpreting it thus. OK, now I think I'm getting it."[11]

When you encounter new information, take charge and reason your way through the learning experience. Make it your goal to have critical thinking pervade your learning practices. Be confident in your ability to learn. Question deeply and use your preferred learning style. Remember, you are your own best teacher.

Memorizing Effectively

As much as experts emphasize that critical thinking is *more* than memorizing (remembering facts), learning how to memorize effectively enhances your ability to think critically: You must be able to recall facts to progress to higher levels of thinking, such as knowing how to apply and analyze information. For example, if you aren't able to *recall* what *normal* health assessment findings are, you won't be able to analyze your patient's data to decide whether there are any *abnormal* findings.

Some disciplines require more memorization than others. Nursing is a discipline that requires a considerable amount of memorization, especially in the beginning. The following strategies are suggested to help you memorize effectively:

1. **Try to understand before you try to memorize.** Once you make sense of the information, you'll begin to realize what's most important and how you can organize it to make remembering easier.
2. **Don't try to memorize everything.** Take the time to identify what's most important; then separate this information from all the other information. This keeps you from trying to memorize too much. Your brain can only take so much new information at a time.

3. **Work to find relationships between the facts, rather than trying to just remember a list of facts.** You can remember *groups of information* easier than isolated facts. The process of trying to understand how the facts relate to each other will also help you *remember* the facts.

4. **Create a memory hook.** Put the information into context. For example, if you've looked after someone with the diagnosis you're studying, visualize the patient and how the situation compares with the information you're studying (the patient then becomes your memory hook). If you don't have a real situation to connect with, play around with the information until something comes to mind that helps you remember (a rhyme, a picture, a story, a mnemonic). For example, consider the following techniques:

   • **Use a mnemonic** (organize what you're trying to remember in such a way that each word's first letter makes a real or nonsensical word).

     Examples:

     TACT helps you remember what you should be monitoring when you're giving medications:

     > **T** = Therapeutic effect
     > **A** = Adverse reactions
     > **C** = Contraindications
     > **T** = Toxicity/overdose

     PERRL (Pupils Equally Round and Reactive to Light) helps you remember to check the pupils to make sure they react equally to light when doing a neurologic assessment.

   • **Use an acrostic** (create a catchy phrase that helps you remember the first letters of the information you're trying to remember).

     Example: **M**aggie **c**hewed **n**uts **e**very **p**lace **s**he **w**ent provides the first letter of things you need to assess when performing a neurovascular assessment: **m**ovement, **c**olor, **n**umbness, **e**dema, **p**ulses, **s**ensation, **w**armth.

5. **In addition to using your preferred learning style, use as many senses as possible.** If you use other senses together with your preferred style, you'll remember even more. For example, use visual and auditory senses together by reading aloud or use all three senses by saying the words as you write and read them.

6. **Organize the information; then see if you can organize it a different way.** By mentally using the information in different ways, you'll remember it better.

BOX 4–8	**Teaching Ourselves: Key Questions**

1. **What major outcomes (observable results) do I/we plan to achieve?** I/we will demonstrate mastery of the required information by passing the appropriate tests or demonstrating competency in real situations.

2. **What problems or issues *must* be addressed to achieve the major outcomes?** Have you clearly identified the knowledge or skills required to pass the test? What's the best way for you to learn this particular information or skill? Do you know test-taking strategies that will help you make educated guesses?

3. **What are the circumstances?** Will you be tested in a real or simulated situation. How important is it for you to pass (e.g., do you get a second chance)? How motivated are you to learn the information or skills?

4. **What knowledge is required?** Required knowledge includes knowledge of self (e.g., preferred learning styles, motivations), learning skills, and critical thinking skills. You must also be clearly aware of the circumstances, as addressed in question 2 above.

5. **How much room is there for error?** Room for error *varies* according to the consequences of what happens if you don't learn the information. For example, in which situation below do you think you have more room for error?
   a. You need to prepare for an open-book exam on nursing care for respiratory problems.
   b. You need to master respiratory assessment and tracheal suctioning before you take care of someone with a tracheostomy tomorrow.
   If you said *a*, you're correct. The risk of harm to your patient leaves little room for error.

6. **How much time do I have?** The time frame for learning depends on when you'll need to use the information. But remember, your brain can only learn so much in one sitting.

7. **What resources can help me?** Human resources include professionals specializing in how to learn, clinical nurse educators, preceptors, clinical nurse specialists, peers, and librarians. Other resources include texts on content, texts on how to learn, articles, computerized learning packages, pamphlets, and audiovisuals.

8. **Whose perspectives must be considered?** The most significant perspective to consider is your *own*. How ready are you to learn? What is it you think you need to learn most? How do you learn best? What usually motivates you to learn? Other perspectives to consider are those of your teachers (e.g., they may be better at teaching one way or another; you need to consider how *they* will know that you've mastered the information or skill.

9. **What's influencing my thinking?** A major influencing factor is whether you *believe* you can master the information or skill (this can be a self-fulfilling prophecy). Thinking may also be influenced by any of the factors listed in Table 2–1, Factors Influencing Critical Thinking Ability (page 30).

7. **Review the information briefly before going to sleep.** Studies show that even if you're a "morning person," information moves into long-term memory better if reviewed late in the day, immediately before going to bed.

8. **Put the information on tape.** Tapes can be played almost anywhere, anytime. Those minutes driving, walking, or riding a bicycle can be valuable time to load information into long-term memory.

9. **Use the information and quiz yourself periodically ("use it or lose it").** Remember, just because you can recognize information in your notes, it doesn't mean you'll be able to *recall* the information *without* your notes.

10. **Know yourself and use self-discipline.** Identify the circumstances that help you retain information and plan your schedule to include those circumstances. For example, if you study better in the morning, be sure you go to bed early enough so that you can get up early and feel rested; if you're easily distracted or sidetracked, plan to go to the library or put a Don't Disturb sign on your door.

To complete this section, review Box 4–8, which answers key critical thinking questions in relation to teaching ourselves.

TEST TAKING

Test taking can be frustrating and anxiety producing. Almost everyone can identify with being in the position of knowing information well yet not being able to perform on the test. Lots of us can reason *well* in real situations but are stumped when it comes to reasoning our way to a correct *test* answer. For example, someone once said to me, "I need a real person and real situation to think well." If you're one of those people (as I am), this section should be helpful to you.

Using critical thinking to identify the best way to prepare for and take tests can reduce your anxiety and improve your test scores. Being successful at test taking requires more than knowledge about the *content*. It also requires that you know yourself, the test format, and test-taking *skills*. The following strategies are suggested to help you improve your test scores:

1. **Know yourself.** Identify your usual test-taking behaviors: For example, Do you get overly anxious? Do you frequently run out of time?

Are you more successful at one type of test than another? Seek help for areas you'd like to change.

2. **Know the test plan.** Find out what types of questions (multiple-choice, short-answer, essay) are going to be asked and what information is most important to study. If the faculty doesn't share this information, review course objectives and text objectives and summaries—often these will help you decide.

3. **Start preparing with an attitude of, I can do this—I just have to figure out how.** You are capable. Sometimes you need to remind yourself of this to acquire the positive attitude we all know is so important.

4. **Get organized and plan ahead.** Decide what you need to study, what your resources are (notes, books, tutors), and when and how you'll prepare for the test.

BOX 4–9	**Components of a Test Question**

1. **The background statement(s).** The statements or phrases that tell you the context in which you're expected to answer the question (e.g., the words in italics below):

   Example Test Question: *You're caring for someone who has severe asthma, is wheezing loudly, is confused, and can't sleep. You check the orders and note that a sedative can be given for sleeplessness.* Knowing the possible effects of giving a sedative to an asthmatic, what would you do?
   a. Give the sedative to help the patient relax.
   b. Withhold the sedative because it aggravates asthma.
   c. Withhold the sedative because it may cause excessive somnolence.
   d. Give the sedative but monitor the patient carefully.

2. **The stem.** A phrase that asks or states the intent of the question. For example, the underlined words above.

3. **Key concepts.** The most important *concepts* addressed in the background statement(s). In the above example the key concepts are severe asthma, wheezing loudly, and effects of giving a sedative to an asthmatic.

4. **Key word(s).** The words that *specify* what's being asked and what's happening. In the example above the key words are "severe," "loudly," and "confused." These words specify that the asthma problem is severe. "Would you do" specifies that you're being asked for an appropriate action to take.

5. **The options (choices).** These include one correct answer (called the *keyed response*) and three to five *distractors* (incorrect answers). In the example above, *c* is the keyed response, and the rest are distractors.

BOX 4–10	**Test Taking: Key Questions**

1. **What major outcomes (observable results) do I plan to achieve?** I will get a (specify grade) on the test.
2. **What problems or issues *must* be addressed to achieve the major outcomes?** Identify (1) what content and skills will be tested, (2) what type of test this will be, and (3) what's the best way for you to prepare for this particular test or situation?
3. **What are the circumstances?** How important is it for you to get your desired score? Will you be tested in real or simulated situations? Do you get a second chance? Are you penalized for guessing?
4. **What knowledge is required?** Required knowledge includes knowledge of the test plan and content and skills to be tested; you also need knowledge of yourself (e.g., study habits, learning style, test-taking patterns).
5. **How much room is there for error?** Room for error *varies* according to the type of test to be taken and the consequences if you don't pass the test.
6. **How much time do I have?** Time frame varies, as we all know!
7. **What resources can help me?** Human resources include professionals specializing in learning and test taking and peers. Other resources include texts and articles on test taking and review books (see Bibliography, page 285).
8. **Whose perspectives must be considered?** Both your own perspective and that of whoever constructed the test must be considered. It's important to realize that the person who is testing you *wants* you to do well but needs to feel comfortable that you've mastered the required content or skills.
9. **What's influencing my thinking?** A major influencing factor is whether you think you can pass the test (this can be a self-fulfilling prophecy). Thinking may also be influenced by any of the factors listed in Table 2–1, Factors Influencing Critical Thinking Ability (page 30).

5. **Learn how to read questions and make educated guesses.** See Boxes 4–9, 4–10, and 4–11.
6. **Practice** answering the types of questions you expect to take on the test (e.g., practice multiple-choice questions for state board exams). One of the reasons some of us don't do well on tests is because we don't take them every day. Often, answering discussion questions and end-of-chapter exercises are also good ways to practice. If you're going to take the test on a computer, practice on the computer. For state board exams, take a review course.
7. **Arrive early for warm-up.** Give yourself time to calm down, get focused, and mentally go through information you've decided is im-

BOX 4–11	**Guidelines for Making Educated Guesses***

Definition: Knowing how to apply test-taking strategies to choose a right answer when you're unsure from content alone (when none of the options seem to jump out at you).

1. Be clear about directions.
2. Find out whether you're penalized for guessing.
3. Read the question **carefully.** Look at *all* the response choices.
   - Eliminate answers you know are outright wrong.
   - Look for answers that are wrong based on the directions.
   - Look for clues in the questions or answers that might help you narrow it down further to the most likely best answer (see strategies 4 and 5 below).
4. When reading test questions, ask yourself four questions:
   - Who is the client? (age, sex, role, etc.)
   - What is the problem? (diagnosis, signs, symptoms, behavior, etc.)
   - What specifically is asked about the problem? (e.g., *To prevent respiratory complications. . . . Because the cast is damp. . . .*)
   - What time frame is being addressed? (e.g., *immediately before surgery, on the day of admission, when?*)
5. Use the following rules *together with your knowledge* to make educated guesses:
   - **Initial = Assessment.** The word *initial* used in a question usually requires an assessment answer. (What would you assess?)
   - **Essential = Safety.** The word *essential* used in a question usually requires a safety answer. (What's required for safety?)
     Remember: "Keep them breathing, keep them safe".
   - **Law of opposites.** If you have two answers that are opposite to one another, the answer is usually *one of these two opposites. Example:* The correct answer is likely to be *a* or *c* below because they're opposites.
     a. Turn the client on the right side.
     b. Encourage fluids.
     c. Turn the client on the left side.
     d. Ambulate the client.

*Strategies provided in consultation with Judith C. Miller, MS RN, President, Nursing Tutorial and Consulting Services, Clifton, VA 20124 1-800-US-TUTOR

BOX 4–11	**Guidelines for Making Educated Guesses** *Continued*

- **Odd man wins.** The option that's most different in length, style, or content is usually the right answer. The right answer is often the longest one or the shortest one. *Example:* The correct answer below is likely to be *b* because it's the "odd man."
  a. Decreased temperature
  b. Rapid pulse
  c. Decreased respirations
  d. Decreased blood pressure
- **Same answer.** If two responses say the same thing in different words, they can't both be right, so neither one is right. *Example: Tachycardia* and *rapid heart beat* as two answer options.
- **Repeated words.** If the answer contains the same word (or a synonym) that appears in the question, it's more likely to be a correct response. *Example:* The word *hypotension* in question, the word *hypotension* or *shock* in answer.
- **Absolutely not.** Answers that use "absolutes" are usually not the right response. *Example: always, never, all, none*
- **Generally so.** Answers that use qualifiers that make the response more "generally so" tend to signify right answers. *Example: usually, frequently, often.*

portant. Reviewing practice questions is also a good way to get your brain in test-taking gear.

8. **If possible, skim the whole test and plan your approach.*** For example, you might begin by answering the types of questions you like before tackling types you don't like (e.g., you may like matching better than essay). Completing what you like and know first reduces anxiety and gets your brain in the test-taking mode before you tackle more difficult questions.

9. **Focus on what you know.**
    - **Skip more difficult questions** and come back to them later.* For example, put a question mark next to questions you *might* be able to answer and an "X" next to the toughest questions. Go back to the question mark questions before the "X" questions.

---

*With some computerized tests, for example, state board exams, you may not be able to move around in the test.

- **For essay tests,** jot down key points you know you want to address before writing your essay. When you're finished, check your essay to be sure you've hit all the major points and that you've been clear.
- **For essay and short-answer questions,** if you have time at the end, come back to these questions and ask yourself, What else can I say? or What did I miss?

10. **Let your instructor know if you don't understand a question.** You may not be allowed to ask questions during the test, but consider writing something like, I wasn't sure if you meant. . . . Or, . . . so I'm answering the question assuming you meant. . . . If allowed, write this on your answer sheet or flip the answer sheet over.

11. **When in doubt, don't change answers.** Studies show your first response is more likely to be correct.

12. **For case history questions,** read questions about the case history first; then read the histories with the intent of looking for the answers.

13. **When you're struggling to answer,** consider whether sketching a picture or diagram will help you conceptualize the answer.

14. **Watch your time and note how the questions are weighted.** For example, if a question is worth 50% of your grade, you might want to save 50% of your time to work on that question.

15. **If you do poorly, don't think it's the end of the world.** Even the brightest, most knowledgeable minds have been known to fail tests (Einstein flunked algebra; Edison was considered unteachable). Instead, *do* something (e.g., explain your difficulty to your instructor; ask if there's some way you can prepare better or if you can do extra credit work; determine resources that can help you; practice, practice, practice).

 OTHER PERSPECTIVES

A Tip for State Board Exams

"I teach students to remember Maslow's hierarchy. . . . 'Keep them breathing, keep them safe.' I had a student who called me to tell me he passed NCLEX. He said what got him through was 'Keep them breathing, keep them safe.'"

—*Judith Miller, MS, RN*
Nursing Tutorial and Consulting Services

SUMMARY

This chapter examines critical thinking in five common nursing concerns: moral and ethical reasoning, nursing research, teaching others, teaching ourselves, and test taking. As health care delivery becomes more complex, you will need sound moral and ethical reasoning skills. Nursing research, required by national practice standards, is essential to improving nursing outcomes. Creative, efficient teaching gives people the knowledge they need to be independent. In this time of rapid changes, we all must know how to identify what we don't know and find ways to learn it. Passing tests requires proper preparation and good test-taking skills.

CRITICAL THINKING EXERCISES

Teaching Others, Teaching Ourselves, Test Taking
1. Explain why knowing how to teach others efficiently is essential to meeting the goals of nursing.*

2. Describe five strategies that can help you memorize more effectively.

3. If you don't know your preferred learning style, study pages 253 and 254 and decide how you best learn.

4. Respond to the following from the prechapter self-test.
   a. Use critical thinking to create a teaching plan. To complete this objective, ask a fellow student something he or she would like to learn and develop a teaching plan using the approaches suggested in this chapter.
   b. Address the roles of memorizing and reasoning in teaching ourselves.*
   c. Describe five strategies that can help you improve your test scores.

---

*An example response for this exercise can be found in the Response Key at the back of the book beginning on page 241.

CRITICAL MOMENTS

The Benefits of Mentors and Role Models
Seek out mentors and role models—teachers, other nurses, friends, and peers. They help you clarify your thoughts and set goals better than any textbook.

Teaching Others Helps You Learn
When you want to know something well, offer to teach it to someone else. You learn and recall best what you teach someone else.

KEY POINTS

- There are seven ethical principles that guide ethical decision making: autonomy, beneficence, justice, fidelity, veracity, confidentiality, and accountability. Practice standards, ethics codes, and bills of rights also guide ethical conduct. Page 105 offers eight key steps for moral and ethical reasoning.

- The following are commonly seen values addressed in ethical codes and standards: maintaining client confidentiality, acting as client advocate, delivering care in a nonjudgmental and nondiscriminatory manner, being sensitive to client diversity and culture, promoting client autonomy, dignity, and rights, and seeking resources for solving ethical dilemmas.

- Advance directives help us make decisions about cardiac resuscitation and other end-of-life treatments.

- Conducting research is one of the most rigorous and disciplined examples of critical thinking in nursing. Research generates knowledge that provides a scientific basis for planning, predicting, and controlling the outcomes of nursing practice.

- Beginning nurses have four main responsibilities in relation to nursing research: (1) to think analytically about the situations they encounter and to seek out research results that might improve nursing care, (2) to raise questions about their practice that might prompt a researcher to formulate a question to guide a study, (3) to help researchers collect data, and (4) to continue to acquire and share knowledge related to research.

- Before you can use research results, you must decide whether the study is valid and reliable (whether it was conducted in such a way that you can trust that the results are accurate).

- Quality Improvement (QI), a responsibility of all nurses, is perhaps the type of research most frequently encountered in the clinical setting. QI studies usually study information from three different perspectives: outcome, process, and structure.

- Because people today are discharged sicker and quicker than they were in the past, we must be able to clearly identify what *must* be learned and then initiate a timely teaching plan that draws on client strengths.

- Today's challenging workplace requires us to identify what it is we must learn and then to find ways to learn it efficiently. Reasoning our way through the learning process helps us connect with our own unique way of making information *ours*.

- Learning how to memorize effectively enhances your ability to think critically: you must be able to recall facts to progress to higher levels of thinking.

- Successful test taking requires that you know yourself, the test format, and test taking skills and how to make an educated guess (see Box 4–11).

Footnotes

[1]From Scanlon, C. (1994, March). Developing ethical competence. *American Nurse*, p. 1.

[2]From Aroskar, M. (1994, March). Ethical decision-making in patient care. *American Nurse*, p. 10.

[3]Jameton, A. (1984). *Nursing practice: The ethical issues.* Englewood Cliffs, NJ: Prentice-Hall.

[4]Summarized from American Nurses Association. (1991). *Standards of clinical nursing practice* (p. 15). Washington, DC: Author.

[5]Taylor, C., Lillis, C., and Lamone, P. (1997). *Fundamentals of nursing: The art and science of nursing care* (3rd ed.). Philadelphia: Lippincott-Raven.

[6]From Burns, N., and Groves, S. (1997). *The practice of nursing research: Conduct, critique, and utilization* (3rd ed., p. 3). Philadelphia: W.B. Saunders Co.

[7]Ibid. p. 4.

[8]Wyoming hospital maps out a better way to care for dying patients. *AACN News*, Feb. 1996, p. 5.

[9]Yutzy, P. (1998). *Hospital of the University of Pennsylvania Alumni Newsletter, 30*(1), p. 5.

[10]Snyder, C. (1998). Humor infusion. *Nursing Spectrum, FL ED, 8*(5), p. 17.

[11]Paul, R. (1993). *Critical thinking: How to prepare students for a rapidly changing world* (p. 305). Santa Rosa, CA: Foundation for Critical Thinking.

See comprehensive bibliography beginning on page 280.

5

Practicing Critical Thinking Skills*: Up Close and Clinical

This chapter at a glance . . .

Read the outcomes listed below and decide whether you can readily achieve each one. If you can, skip this chapter. If you can achieve only some of the outcomes, complete only the sections you need to practice.

LEARNING OUTCOMES

After studying this chapter, you should be able to:

- Explain why each skill in this section promotes critical thinking (see This Chapter at a Glance).

- Explain how to accomplish each skill in this section.

- Be explicit about your thinking in various simulated clinical situations (clearly express how you came to a conclusion or made a decision).

- Identify five critical thinking skills you'd like to improve.

---

*The names and definitions of some of the skills in this section are slightly different from those listed in Chapter 3 (page 48). This is because some of the skills are addressed in more detail in this section, and some of the skills are combined to facilitate learning the skills within the framework of the nursing process.

†This skill deals with identifying risk factors *in healthy people*; the next skill deals with risk factors in the context of people with *existing health problems.*

ABSTRACT

This chapter provides opportunities to practice critical thinking skills in simulated nursing situations based on real experiences. Organized in logical progression according to how the skills might be used in the nursing process, each skill is presented in the following format: (1) Name of the skill, (2) definition of the skill, (3) why the skill promotes critical thinking, (4) how to accomplish the skill, and (5) practice exercises.

CRITICAL THINKING SKILLS: DYNAMIC AND INTERRELATED

Each skill in this section is presented as a *separate* skill. However, these skills aren't usually used *separately* or necessarily at any one particular point in thinking. Your mind thinks in a much more dynamic and rapid way than can be described in a book, often combining skills and moving back and forth between them before coming to a conclusion.

Many of these skills depend on and facilitate one another. For example, you may be giving nursing care and *recognize inconsistencies* (skill 8) in how the person is responding. Recognizing inconsistencies may trigger you to think, *Have I identified assumptions?* (skill 1).

WHAT'S THE POINT?

Just as tennis players break down interrelated tennis skills (stroke, foot placement, ball placement, etc.) into parts to analyze and improve their games *as a whole,* this section breaks down interrelated intellectual skills into parts to help you to analyze and improve your thinking *as a whole.*

To keep the length of this chapter manageable, this section focuses mainly on critical thinking in the context of *problems.* However, keep in mind that using critical thinking also requires you to look for ways to improve areas that *are satisfactory* but could be better.

GENERAL INSTRUCTIONS

1. **To get the most out of these exercises, don't try to do too many at one time.** Some of these exercises, as in real life, are quite time consuming. The purpose of the exercises *isn't* to do them as quickly as possible. Rather, take your time and get in touch with your thinking as you do them. If possible, get at least one other person to complete the exercises with you. You'll learn more by discussing the skills with others.

2. **Your brain is a tricky thing—describing what goes on in someone's head to accomplish these skills is difficult.** If you're having trouble with a section, read on and come back to it later. Subsequent sections and skills are likely to help you clarify questions. Doing the practice exercises will also help you clarify the skill.

3. **If you encounter a disease or drug that you don't know, look it up.** As stated earlier, critical thinking in nursing requires knowledge of problem-specific facts (see Box 3–9, page 89). Looking up the disease or drug and *applying* the information to the exercise will help you build your own mental storehouse of problem-specific facts. You remember best information that you *use.*

4. **Before starting this section, be sure you master the following vocabulary.** These terms are listed in order of how they can best be learned (you need to know the first term to understand the second term, and so on).

REQUIRED VOCABULARY FOR COMPLETING THIS CHAPTER

Definitive Diagnosis. The most *specific,* most correct diagnosis. For example, someone may be admitted with an initial diagnosis of respiratory distress. Then, after studies are completed, it may be decided that the definitive diagnosis is *congestive heart failure.* To identify the *best interventions* (actions), you must determine the *most specific diagnosis.*

Causative Factor. Something known to make a problem happen. For example, a high blood level of uric acid is known to cause gout.

Risk Factor. Something known to be associated with a specific problem. For example, having a family history of gout is a *risk factor* for gout. The terms *causative factor* and *risk factor* are often used interchangeably.

Related Factor. See Risk Factor.

Potential Problem or Risk Diagnosis. A problem or diagnosis that may occur because of certain risk or causative factors present. For example, someone who's on prolonged bed rest has a potential or risk for Impaired Skin Integrity. Often used interchangeably with *high-risk problem or diagnosis.*

Data. Pieces of information about health status (for example, vital signs).

Objective Data. Information that you can clearly observe or measure (for example, a pulse of 140 beats per minute). To remember this term, remember:

O-O = Objective data are Observed

Subjective Data. Information the patient states or communicates. Often these are the patient's *perceptions.* For example, "My heart feels like it's racing." To remember this term, remember:

S-S = Subjective data are Stated (or written or signed in sign language)

Cues. Synonymous with *data.* Often used interchangeably with *signs and symptoms.*

Signs and Symptoms. Abnormal data that prompt you to suspect a health problem. *Signs* refer to objective data. *Symptoms* refer to subjective data. *Examples:* Fever is a sign of infection; chest pain is a symptom of heart disease.

Defining Characteristics. Signs and symptoms usually present with a diagnosis.

Baseline Data. Data collected before treatment begins. May also refer to data that represents the patient's usual state.

Data Base Assessment. Comprehensive data collection performed to gain comprehensive information about *all* aspects of health status (e.g., respiratory status, neurologic status, circulatory status, and so on).

Focus Assessment. Data collection that aims to gain specific (focused) information about only *one* aspect of health status (e.g., neurologic status).

Infer. To suspect something or to attach meaning to a cue. For example, if an infant doesn't stop crying, no matter what's done for him, you might infer that *he's in pain.*

Inference. Something we suspect to be true, based on a logical conclusion. For example, the italicized words above.

MPRC. A mnemonic that stands for Monitor, Prevent, Resolve, and Control. A plan of care should *monitor, prevent, resolve,* and *control* problems.

1. IDENTIFYING ASSUMPTIONS

Definition

Recognizing information taken for granted or presented as fact without evidence. For example, we might assume a woman on a maternity unit has just had a baby.

Why This Skill Promotes Critical Thinking

Critical thinking aims to make judgments based on evidence. If we reason based on assumptions, our thinking is likely to be flawed. By recognizing our assumptions, we can overcome our natural tendency to take things for granted, and get the *facts,* before going on to identify problems and make decisions.

Guidelines: How to Accomplish This Skill

The best way to identify assumptions is to *look* for them. Whenever making any important decisions, before you make a plan of action, ask questions like, What's being taken for granted here? and How do I know that I've got the facts right? Other skills that follow will also help you identify assumptions.

Practice Exercises: Identifying Assumptions

Example responses are on pages 241 and 242.

1. Explain why the following statement is an assumption: *We've got to*

teach this patient how to stick to a low-salt diet because he eats whatever he wants even though his doctor told him not to eat salt.

2. What could happen if you planned nursing care based on the preceding assumption?

3. Read the following scenarios; then answer the questions that follow them.

Scenario One

Anita's plan today is to teach Jeff about diabetes. She's well prepared and decides she'll create a positive attitude for Jeff by telling him about all the advances in diabetic care. She doesn't have much time, so she introduces herself and starts telling him how much easier it is to manage diabetes than it used to be. She goes on to explain how easy it can be to learn the required diet, monitor blood sugar at home, and take insulin. Jeff listens to all Anita has to say, asks a few questions, then leaves with his wife. As they drive off, he says to his wife in a discouraged tone, "She sure is a know-it-all, isn't she?"

a. Based on the information provided, what assumption does it seem Anita made about creating a positive attitude?

b. What key thing did Anita forget to do that might have helped her avoid making this assumption?

c. Why do you think Jeff said Anita was a know-it-all?

Scenario Two

Four-year-old Bobby is in the emergency department with his mother. He fell off his bike and had an initial period of unconsciousness lasting about a minute. He's been examined, has no skull fracture, and is now awake and alert, ready to go home with his mother. The nurse gives his mother a computer printout of instructions for checking Bobby's neurologic status at home and says, "Let me know if you have questions."

a. What assumption does it seem the nurse has made?

b. What might happen if the nurse's assumption is incorrect?

Scenario Three

A friend of mine told me this story:

I had just started working evenings in the emergency department of a seaside town hospital. We admitted a 54-year-old man, whom I'll call Mr. Schmidt. Mr. Schmidt told me, "I just got here for vacation, and I'm not feeling so great. I had pneumonia at home, got treated, and thought I was better. Now my breathing feels lousy again." A check of his vital signs while he was sitting quietly revealed the following: T 99 P 138 R 36 BP 168/80.

As I helped him to the stretcher, he became significantly more short of breath. I checked his lung sounds and heard a lot of congestion. I notified the physician and voiced my concern that Mr. Schmidt seemed quite ill. The doctor immediately examined him and ordered an EKG and chest x-ray.

During this time we got very busy. I was helping another patient when the physician came to me and said, "I want you to give Mr. Schmidt 80 mg of furosemide (a diuretic) IV now and discharge him."

I looked at him skeptically and said, "*Discharge* him?"

He said, "Yes. I'm sure the diuretic will help him get rid of this fluid."

Being new and not really knowing this physician, I tried to tactfully voice my concern about this idea. "Can we give him some time to see how he responds?"

"Nope. This place is wild. I'm sending him home. He's going to a private physician in the morning. He'll be fine once he gets rid of some fluid. Discharge him with instructions to call if he doesn't feel better."

Reluctantly, I went to give Mr. Schmidt the furosemide. I still had trouble with the idea of sending this man home before knowing his response to the IV diuretic.

Then I decided to use my own clout as a nurse: I had established a rapport with the Schmidts, and they trusted me. Before I gave the drug, I said, "I realize the doctor has discharged you, but I'd be interested to see if there's any change in blood pressure after you get rid of some fluid. How would you feel about sitting in the waiting room, and I'll check your blood pressure in an hour?" Both the Schmidts thought this was a good idea and went off to the waiting room. Only 45 minutes had passed when there was a shout for help. I ran to the waiting room and found Mr. Schmidt on the floor having a grand mal seizure. He then stopped breathing.

We were able to resuscitate Mr. Schmidt, and he was admitted to the hospital, diagnosed with electrolyte imbalance and heart failure, and discharged a week later.

a. What assumption does it seem the physician made about Mr. Schmidt's response to the furosemide?
b. Why do you think the nurse was so concerned about the assumption the physician made?
c. What assumption does it seem the nurse made about how the physician would respond to her if she cautioned him about discharging Mr. Schmidt?

 OTHER PERSPECTIVES

Avoiding Making Assumptions
"Heightened awareness often precedes a change in behavior. For example, once you know you tend to make assumptions, you soon begin to double-check your thinking."

—*Carol Matz, RN, MSN, Nursing Faculty*

2. IDENTIFYING AN ORGANIZED AND COMPREHENSIVE APPROACH TO DISCOVERY (ASSESSMENT)

Definition

Choosing a systematic approach that enhances the ability to discover *all* the information needed to fully understand someone's health status.

Why This Skill Promotes Critical Thinking

One of the leading causes of critical thinking errors is making judgments or decisions based on incomplete information. Having a well thought out, organized approach to assessment prevents you from forgetting something. For example, if you're interrupted while performing a physical assessment, you know exactly where you left off and where to continue. If you consistently use the same organized approach, you also form *habits* that help you be systematic and complete.

Guidelines: How to Accomplish This Skill

How you organize your assessment depends on the patient's health status:

- **If the person is acutely ill,** set immediate priorities by using an approach such as the ABC's and the MAA-U-AR approach listed in Box 3–10, page 91.
- **If the person has a specific problem,** begin by assessing *the problem* first; then go on to complete the assessment in the same way you would if the person were healthy.
- **If the person is generally healthy,** choose any organized method you find convenient. For example, use the head-to-toe approach, the body systems approach (Fig. 3–3, page 80), the functional health patterns approach (Box 3–5, page 80), or follow a preprinted assessment tool (see example, Fig. 5–1, page 146).

Critical Thinking and Preestablished Assessment Tools. Most facilities have developed assessment tools that nurses are required to complete for each patient. Some of these tools are designed for *data base assessment* (see example, page 146), and others are designed for *focus assessment* (see example, page 149). If you'd like to see an example of what these assessment tools look like when they're completed by a nurse, check pages 258 to 263 (Appendix D).

While preestablished assessment tools can help you develop habits that promote an organized and comprehensive approach to assessment, you must use these guides appropriately:

- Before using a tool, determine why the information the tool guides you to collect is *relevant.* For example, suppose you use the neurologic assessment tool on page 149, and you're collecting data about how the pupils react to light. Find out *why this information is relevant* to determining neurologic status. To move more quickly toward an expert level of thinking, make the connection between what information is requested and *why* it's relevant.
- Remember the importance of gathering both subjective data (patient's perceptions) and objective data (your observations).
- Keep in mind that assessment tools don't prompt you to use all your resources. After you interview and examine your patient, ask, What other resources might provide additional information about this person's health status (medical and nursing records, significant others, other health care professionals)?

To become skilled at identifying an organized and comprehensive approach to assessment:

1. Choose a method of assessment and use it consistently.
2. Locate assessment tools that are designed for your patient's specific situation, practice using them, and be sure you understand why you collect each piece of data.
3. Keep in mind that a body systems approach to assessment helps you collect data about *medical problems.* Nursing models, such as functional health patterns, help you collect data about *nursing problems.*

Practice Exercises: Identifying an Organized and Comprehensive Approach to Discovery (Assessment)

Example responses are on pages 242 to 244.

1. You're working as a school nurse and have been asked to perform physical exams to screen students for possible medical problems before they see the doctor. Identify an organized, comprehensive approach to assessing for signs and symptoms of a medical problem.

2. You're making a home visit to Mrs. Sossa, who has a newborn child and seven other children under 12 years old. Both the baby and the mother are healthy. Identify an organized and comprehensive approach to assessing for problems with human responses.

3. Read the following scenarios; then answer the questions that follow them.

Scenario One

Pearl, an 89-year-old grandmother, is admitted overnight after fracturing her left ankle. She had surgery and a cast applied today. The cast goes from her toes to below the knee. Her toes are visible, and she can wiggle them freely. A small window has been cut in the cast over the dorsalis pedis pulse. Routine hospital protocols state that anyone with a new cast must have neurovascular checks every 2 hours for the first day of hospitalization. You know the following acrostic helps you remember the things you need to check when performing a neurovascular assessment for someone with a cast: **M**aggie **C**hewed **N**uts **E**very **P**lace **S**he **W**ent stands for:
Movement, **C**olor, **N**umbness, **E**dema, **P**ulses, **S**ensation, **W**armth

a. Using the preceding acrostic to help you assess systematically, how would you assess to determine the neurovascular status of Pearl's injured leg?
b. Why is it necessary to monitor each of the above assessment parameters to determine neurovascular status?
c. What would you do if Pearl told you her toes felt numb and cold?

Scenario Two

You're about to give Mr. Wu digoxin by mouth. You know that the mnemonic TACT helps you remember what you need to assess to monitor responses to medications and determine whether there are any reasons to withhold them:
T = **Therapeutic effect** (Is there a *therapeutic effect*?)
A = **Adverse reactions** (Are there signs of *adverse reactions*?)
C = **Contraindications** (Are there any *contraindications* to giving this drug?)
T = **Toxicity/overdose** (Are there signs of *toxicity or overdose*?)
   Using **TACT** to focus your assessment to systematically gather information about how Mr. Wu is responding to the digoxin:

a. How would you assess him to decide whether to give the digoxin?
b. Why is it important to determine all of the things listed in the mnemonic **TACT**?

Scenario Three

You just admitted Gerome, who fell off his bike, hit his head, and had a short period of unconsciousness. He is now awake and alert but is admitted for 24 hours of neurologic monitoring. The physician orders neurologic assessments every hour.

Respond to the questions that follow, using the neurologic focus assessment guide that follows the questions.

a. How would you assess Gerome to determine the status of each of the neurologic assessment parameters addressed in the guide?
b. Why is each piece of data on the focus assessment guide relevant to determining neurologic status?
c. What would you do if, on admission, Gerome demonstrates normal neurologic assessment findings but 2 hours later demonstrates extreme drowsiness (he awakens only if you shake him and call his name)?
d. What would you do if one pupil started to become more sluggish in its response to light than the other?
e. What would you do if you noted a general pattern of the pulse getting slower than baseline pulse?

Neurologic Focus Assessment Guide

VITAL SIGNS   Temp._____   Pulse_____   Resp._____   BP_____

(Place a check mark in front of words that apply)

EYE OPENING
☐ Spontaneous   ☐ To command   ☐ To pain   ☐ No response

BEST MOTOR RESPONSE
☐ Obeys commands   ☐ Localizes pain   ☐ Flexion withdrawal
☐ Abnormal flexion   ☐ Abnormal extension   ☐ No response

BEST VERBAL RESPONSE
☐ Oriented   ☐ Confused   ☐ Inappropriate words
☐ Incomprehensible words   ☐ No response

PUPIL REACTION
Right eye: _____Size of pupil   _____Reaction to light (brisk, sluggish)
Left eye: _____Size of pupil   _____Reaction to light (brisk, sluggish)

PURPOSEFUL LIMB MOVEMENT

Right arm
☐ Spontaneous   ☐ To command   ☐ Paralysis
☐ Visible muscle contraction but no movement
☐ Weak contraction; not enough to overcome gravity
☐ Moves against gravity, not to external resistance
☐ Normal range of motion; can be overcome by increased gravity
☐ Normal muscle strength

Right leg
☐ Spontaneous   ☐ To command   ☐ Paralysis
☐ Visible muscle contraction but no movement
☐ Weak contraction; not enough to overcome gravity
☐ Moves against gravity, not to external resistance
☐ Normal range of motion; can be overcome by increased gravity
☐ Normal muscle strength

Left arm
☐ Spontaneous   ☐ To command   ☐ Paralysis
☐ Visible muscle contraction but no movement
☐ Weak contraction; not enough to overcome gravity
☐ Moves against gravity, not to external resistance
☐ Normal range of motion; can be overcome by increased gravity
☐ Normal muscle strength

Left leg
☐ Spontaneous   ☐ To command   ☐ Paralysis
☐ Visible muscle contraction but no movement
☐ Weak contraction; not enough to overcome gravity
☐ Moves against gravity, not to external resistance
☐ Normal range of motion; can be overcome by increased gravity
☐ Normal muscle strength

LIMB SENSATION (PRICK LIMB WITH STERILE NEEDLE)
Right arm: ☐ Normal   ☐ Decreased   ☐ Absent
Right leg: ☐ Normal   ☐ Decreased   ☐ Absent
Left arm: ☐ Normal   ☐ Decreased   ☐ Absent
Left leg: ☐ Normal   ☐ Decreased   ☐ Absent

SEIZURE ACTIVITY: Describe in nurse's notes.

GAG REFLEX: ☐ Present   ☐ Absent

NURSING ADMISSION ASSESSMENT

DATE _____ TIME OF ARRIVAL _____

FROM _____

ACCOMPANIED BY _____

VIA: WHEELCHAIR _____ STRETCHER _____ AMBULATORY _____

ID BRACELET _____ INFORMATION OBTAINED FROM _____

I. VITAL STATISTICS

   TEMP _____ PULSE _____ RESP _____

   ORAL _____ RECTAL _____ AXILLARY _____

   BP _____ RA _____ LA _____ POSITION _____

   WEIGHT _____ HEIGHT _____

   SCALE: BED _____ CHAIR _____ STANDING _____

   DEFERRED _____

   ORIENTED TO ROOM _____

PROSTHESIS, APPLIANCES OR OTHER DEVICES:

DENTURES ____   *WALKER/CANE/CRUTCHES __

FULL: UPPER ____ LOWER ____   *ARTIFICIAL LIMBS ____

PARTIAL: UPPER ____ LOWER ____   *BRACES ____

EYE GLASSES ____   *FALSE EYE ____

CONTACT LENSES ____   WIG ____

HEARING AID ____

OTHER _____

COMMENTS _____

PATIENT HAS BROUGHT TO HOSPITAL? YES ____ NO ____

EXCEPTIONS _____

II. ALLERGIES: DRUGS _____ DYES _____ FOOD _____ OTHER _____ NONE KNOWN _____

SPECIFY AGENT	DESCRIBE REACTION (IF KNOWN)

III. HEALTH PERCEPTION-HEALTH MAINTENANCE

  A. PRESENT ILLNESS:

     1. ADMITTING DIAGNOSIS _____

     2. REASON FOR ADMISSION (PATIENT'S STATEMENT) _____

     3. DURATION OF PRESENT ILLNESS _____

     4. PAST AND PRESENT TREATMENT OF PRESENT ILLNESS AND RESPONSE _____

     5. PATIENT AWARE OF DIAGNOSIS: YES _____ NO _____ NOT ESTABLISHED _____

  B. PREVIOUS ILLNESSES: (INCLUDING HOSPITALIZATION)

     _____

     _____

8183 PG 1 (REV 9/90)

FIGURE 5–1

Assessment tools are reprinted with permission of the Bryn Mawr Hospital, Bryn Mawr, Pennsylvania.

Figure continued on following pages

C. ARE YOU TAKING ANY MEDICATIONS (PRESCRIBED OR OVER THE COUNTER) YES _____ NO _____

MEDICATION	DOSE	WHEN DO YOU TAKE IT	WHY DO YOU TAKE IT	LAST DOSE	BROUGHT TO HOSPITAL		DISPOSITION
					YES	NO	

D. DO YOU OR HAVE YOU EVER USED?

	YES	NO	LAST USED	FREQUENCY/AMOUNT
ALCOHOL				
RECREATIONAL DRUGS				

E. DO YOU SMOKE? YES _____ PKS/DAY _____ HOW LONG _____

         NO: DID YOU EVER SMOKE? NO ____ YES ____ PKS/DAY _____ HOW LONG _____ WHEN DID YOU QUIT _____

IV. COGNITIVE PERCEPTUAL: HEADACHE _____ SEIZURES _____ BLACKOUTS _____ DIZZINESS _____ NO C/O _____

A. LEVEL OF CONSCIOUSNESS: ALERT _____ DROWSY _____ RESPONDS TO: PAIN _____ VERBAL STIMULI _____ UNRESPONSIVE _____

B. ORIENTED: TIME _____ PLACE _____ PERSON _____ COMMENTS _____

C. MOOD: RELAXED _____ ANXIOUS _____ SAD _____ ANGRY _____ WITHDRAWN _____ OTHER_____

D. RECENT MEMORY CHANGE: YES _____ NO _____ SPECIFY_____

E. RESPONDS TO DIRECTIONS: YES _____ NO _____ SPECIFY_____

F. SPEECH: CLEAR _____ SLURRED _____ GARBLED _____ UNABLE TO SPEAK _____ APHASIC_____

G. LANGUAGE SPOKEN: ENGLISH _____ OTHER _____

H. HEARING: WNL _____ IMPAIRED _____ CORRECTED _____ DEAF _____ SIGN LANGUAGE _____ LIP READS _____

I. VISION: WNL _____ IMPAIRED _____ CORRECTED _____ BLIND _____

J. PAIN: YES _____ NO _____ DESCRIBE _____

     HOW DO YOU MANAGE YOUR PAIN? _____

K. LEARNING READINESS: NO LIMITATIONS _____ WILLING TO LEARN _____ RESISTS LEARNING _____

     EMOTIONALLY READY TO LEARN: YES _____ NO _____ REQUIRES CONCRETE LANGUAGE/REINFORCEMENT _____ FORGETFUL _____

     TEACHING TO BE DIRECTED PRIMARILY TO _____
                                       FAMILY MEMBER/SIGNIFICANT OTHER

L. COMMENTS _____

V. ROLE RELATIONSHIP (PSYCHOSOCIAL) / DISCHARGE PLANNING

A. OCCUPATION _____

B. LIVE ALONE _____ WITH FAMILY _____ NURSING HOME _____ OTHER _____ COMMENT _____

C. DESCRIBE PHYSICAL ENVIRONMENT _____

D. ANTICIPATED DISCHARGE TO: ECF _____ HOME CARE SERVICES _____

     OTHER _____ HOME _____ IF GOING HOME, WHO COULD HELP YOU WITH

     HEALTHCARE NEEDS AFTER DISCHARGE? _____

E. DO YOU WISH TO SEE A MEMBER OF THE CLERGY WHILE YOU ARE HERE? YES _____ NO _____ AFFILIATION_____

F. COMMENTS_____

VI. HEALTH HISTORY/ASSESSMENT

A. CARDIOVASCULAR: ANGINA _____ ARRHYTHMIA _____ MURMUR _____ EDEMA _____ PALPITATIONS _____

     CHEST PAIN _____ MI _____ CVA _____ ANEURYSM _____ HYPERTENSION _____

     PACEMAKER _____ TYPE _____ NO C/O _____

     PULSE: STRONG _____ WEAK _____ REGULAR _____ IRREGULAR _____

     RIGHT DORSALIS.PEDAL PULSE: STRONG _____ WEAK _____ ABSENT _____

     LEFT DORSALIS PEDAL PULSE: STRONG _____ WEAK _____ ABSENT _____

     COMMENTS_____

8183 PG 2 (REV 9/90)

FIGURE 5-1

Continued

B. RESPIRATORY: COUGH _____ PRODUCTIVE _____ PAIN _____ DESCRIBE _____

FREQUENT COLDS ____ HOARSENESS ____ ASTHMA ____ TB ____ SOB: ON EXERTION ____ AT REST ____ NO C/O ____

COMMENTS _____

_____

C. RENAL: KIDNEY STONES ____ INFECTIONS ____ RETENTION ____ BURNING ____ POLYURIA ____ DYSURIA ____ NO C/O ____

URINARY DEVICES? _____ TYPE _____

INCONTINENCE _____ DAYTME _____ NOCTURNAL _____ STRESS _____

DO YOU GET UP DURING NIGHT TO URINATE? YES _____ NO _____

COMMENTS _____

_____

D. GASTROINTESTINAL (NUTRITION/METABOLIC)

1. HISTORY OF DIABETES? YES ____ NO ____ DO YOU TEST FOR SUGAR? YES ____ NO ____ URINE ____ BLOOD ____

DIET CONTROLLED _____ INSULIN DEPENDENT _____ ORAL HYPOGLYCEMICS _____

NUMBER OF YEARS _____ PREVIOUS DIABETES EDUCATION: YES _____ NO _____

2. NUMBER OF MEALS/DAY _____ SNACKS _____ SPECIAL DIET _____

3. PATIENT'S ABILITY TO EAT: INDEPENDENT _____ WITH ASSISTANCE _____ SPECIFY _____

DIFFICULTY SWALLOWING _____

4. WEIGHT CHANGE IN THE LAST SIX MONTHS: NONE _____ LOST _____ LBS GAINED _____ LBS

5. DO YOU EXPERIENCE NAUSEA/VOMITING? YES _____ NO _____ RELATED TO _____

6. DO YOU EXPERIENCE CRAMPING _____ HEARTBURN _____ RECTAL PAIN _____ GAS _____ LAST BM: _____

7. BOWEL: USUAL TIME: _____ A.M. _____ P.M. FREQUENCY: DAILY _____ EVERY OTHER DAY _____ OTHER _____

INCONTINENCE _____ DEVICES USED _____

COLOR: BROWN _____ CLAY-COLORED _____ BLACK _____ BLOOD _____

CONSTIPATION: NONE _____ OCCASIONALLY _____ FREQUENTY _____

DIARRHEA: NONE _____ OCCASIONALLY _____ FREQUENTLY _____ OSTOMY _____

LAXATIVES/ENEMAS USED/HOW OFTEN? (SPECIFY) _____

8. ABDOMEN: SOFT _____ NON-TENDER _____ NON-DISTENDED _____ FIRM _____ TENDER _____ DISTENDED _____

BOWEL SOUNDS: PRESENT _____ ABSENT _____

COMMENTS: _____

_____

E. SKIN CONDITION

COLOR: WNL _____ PALE _____ CYANOTIC _____ JAUNDICE _____ OTHER _____

TEMP: WARM _____ COOL _____ TURGOR: WNL _____ POOR _____

EDEMA: NO _____ YES _____ DESCRIPTION/LOCATION _____

LESIONS: NO _____ YES _____ DESCRIPTION/LOCATION _____

DECUBITUS: NO _____ YES _____ LOCATION(S) _____ (SEE TISSUE TRAUMA FORM)

BRUISES: NO _____ YES _____ DESCRIPTION/LOCATION _____

RASHES: NO _____ YES _____ DESCRIPTION/LOCATION _____

REDNESS: NO _____ YES _____ DESCRIPTION/LOCATION _____

COMMENTS: _____

_____

8183 PG 3 (REV 9/90)

FIGURE 5–1

Continued

F. MUSCULO-SKELETAL: CRAMPING _____ ARTHRITIS _____ STIFFNESS _____ SWELLING _____ NO C/O _____

MOTOR FUNCTION: RIGHT ARM: WNL ____ AMPUTATED ____ SPASTIC ____ FLACCID ____ WEAKNESS ____ PARALYSIS ____ OTHER ____

LEFT ARM: WNL ____ AMPUTATED ____ SPASTIC ____ FLACCID ____ WEAKNESS ____ PARALYSIS ____ OTHER ____

RIGHT LEG: WNL ____ AMPUTATED ____ SPASTIC ____ FLACCID ____ WEAKNESS ____ PARALYSIS ____ OTHER ____

LEFT LEG: WNL ____ AMPUTATED ____ SPASTIC ____ FLACCID ____ WEAKNESS ____ PARALYSIS ____ OTHER ____

COMMENTS _____

_____

VII. SLEEP-REST/ACTIVITY

A. USUAL SLEEP PATTERN: BEDTIME _____ HOURS SLEPT _____ NAPS: NO _____ YES _____

B. DIFFICULTY FALLING ASLEEP: NO _____ YES _____ SPECIFY _____

C. SLEEP AIDS USED: NO _____ YES _____ SPECIFY _____

D. DOES PATIENT HAVE DIFFICULTY/PROBLEMS IN:

BATHING: NO _____ YES _____ SPECIFY _____

DRESSING: NO _____ YES _____ SPECIFY _____

AMBULATING: NO _____ YES _____ BALANCE/GAIT: STEADY _____ UNSTEADY _____ TIRES EASILY _____ WEAKNESS _____

COMMENTS _____

VIII. SEXUAL HEALTH (FEMALES)

A. LMP _____ LAST PAP SMEAR _____

B. DO YOU EXAMINE YOUR BREASTS? YES _____ NO _____ HOW OFTEN? _____

C. IF NO, DO YOU KNOW HOW? YES _____ NO _____ WOULD YOU BE INTERESTED IN LEARNING? YES _____ NO _____

PAMPHLET GIVEN? YES _____ NO _____ COMMENTS _____

IX. ASSESSMENT SUMMARY: _____

_____

_____

X. NURSING DIAGNOSES: _____

_____

_____

_____

_____

XI. THE FOLLOWING SECTIONS WERE DEFERRED ON ADMISSION (IDENTIFY BY SECTION NUMBER): _____

_____

REASON: _____

DATE/TIME	COMPLETED BY		PRIMARY NURSE	DATE/TIME	REVIEWED BY PRIMARY NURSE	
_____/_____	_____	RN	YES ____ NO ____	_____/_____	_____	RN
_____/_____	_____	RN	YES ____ NO ____	_____/_____	_____	RN

8183 PG 4 (REV 9/90)

FIGURE 5–1

Continued

THE BRYN MAWR HOSPITAL NURSING DEPARTMENT

NEUROLOGICAL ASSESSMENT SHEET

Pupil size reference circles: 1MM 2MM 3MM 4MM 5MM 6MM 7MM 8MM 9MM

	DATE														
	TIME														
VITALS	BLOOD PRESSURE														RESPIRATORY TYPE
	PULSE														N = NORMAL
	TEMPERATURE														CS = CHEYNE STOKES
	RESPIRATORY RATE														SH = SUSTAINED HYPERVENTILATION
	RESPIRATORY TYPE														

COMA SCALE

EYES OPEN	SPONTANEOUSLY	4												E = EYES CLOSED BY SWELLING
	TO COMMAND	3												
	TO PAIN	2												
	NO RESPONSE	1												
BEST MOTOR RESPONSE	OBEYS COMMANDS	6												RECORD BEST ARM RESPONSE
	LOCALIZES PAIN	5												
	FLEXION WITHDRAWAL	4												
	FLEXION (ABNORMAL)	3												
	EXTENSION (ABNORMAL)	2												
	NO RESPONSE	1												
BEST VERBAL RESPONSE	ORIENTED	5												T = ENDOTRACHEAL TUBE OR TRACHEOSTOMY
	CONFUSED	4												
	INAPPROPRIATE WORDS	3												
	INCOMPREHENSIBLE SOUNDS	2												A = APHASIA
	NO RESPONSE	1												
	TOTAL SCORE														

PUPILS

SIZE	R													B = BRISK, S = SLUGGISH, N = NO REACTION, C = CLOSED, SC = SUSTAINED CONSTRICTION 2° CATARACT SURGERY
REACTION														
SIZE	L													
REACTION														

LIMB MOVEMENT

GRADE LIMB SPONTANEOUS OR TO COMMAND. DO NOT RATE REFLEX MOVEMENT														LIMB MOVEMENT SCALE
	RA													0 = PARALYSIS
	RL													1 = VISIBLE MUSCLE CONTRACTION; NO MOVEMENT
	LA													2 = WEAK CONTRACTION; NOT ENOUGH TO OVERCOME GRAVITY
	LL													3 = MOVE AGAINST GRAVITY; NOT EXTERNAL RESISTANCE

LIMB SENSATION

DULL	RA													4 = NORMAL ROM; CAN BE OVERCOME BY INCREASED GRAVITY
	RL													5 = NORMAL MUSCLE STRENGTH
	LA													SENSATION CODES
	LL													N = NORMAL
SHARP	RA													D = DECREASED
	RL													A = ABSENT
	LA													
	LL													

SEIZURE ACTIVITY														A = ABSENT, P = PRESENT
GAG REFLEX														A = ABSENT, P = PRESENT
INITIALS														

SIGNATURE	INITIALS	SIGNATURE	INITIALS

F8084
(REV. 1/91)

FIGURE 5–2

Assessment tools are reprinted with permission of the Bryn Mawr Hospital, Bryn Mawr, Pennsylvania.

149

3. CHECKING ACCURACY AND RELIABILITY OF DATA (VALIDATION)

Definition

Verifying information to determine if it's factual.

Why This Skill Promotes Critical Thinking

Critical thinking aims to make judgments based on evidence. You must double check to be sure your information is accurate, factual, and complete. If you don't, you may make decisions based on incorrect or incomplete information. Checking accuracy and reliability also promotes *comprehensive data collection* because it requires you to gather more data to double-check whether you've been correct.

Guidelines: How to Accomplish This Skill

To check accuracy and reliability, review the data already gathered and ask, What data might need verifying here? Then focus your assessment to gain more information to verify or negate that information. For example, an elderly person may have told you that she took her medicine. To verify this, interview significant others or caregivers or check previous records.

Practice Exercises: Checking Accuracy and Reliability of Data (Validation)

Example responses are on page 244.

For each of the following, determine how you would validate whether the data are accurate and reliable:

1. The off-going nurse tells you that Mrs. Molinas is depressed and angry about being in the hospital.
2. Mr. Nola tells you he thinks his blood sugar was about 104 when he tested it an hour ago.
3. You take a blood pressure from the left arm and find it to be abnormally high.
4. Mr. McGwire's care plan states that he has *Knowledge Deficit: Diabetic foot care as evidenced by frequent foot ulcers.*

4. DISTINGUISHING NORMAL FROM ABNORMAL/IDENTIFYING SIGNS AND SYMPTOMS

Definition

Determining what data are *within* normal range and what data are *outside* the usual range for normalcy. Abnormal data are considered signs, symptoms, or cues of a possible problem.

Example: If a 62-year-old man who is taking no medications has a pulse of 42 beats per minute, you know that this is *abnormal*. It may be a sign of a medical problem because a normal pulse rate rarely drops below 55 to 60 beats per minute in someone this age who takes no medications (some cardiac medications lower the heart rate).

Why This Skill Promotes Critical Thinking

Recognizing abnormal data (signs and symptoms) is the first step to problem identification: Signs and symptoms are like red flags that prompt you to suspect a health problem. If you miss red flags, you miss recognizing possible problems.

Guidelines: How to Accomplish This Skill

Identifying signs and symptoms requires that you apply knowledge of what are considered normal findings. This skill also requires using your senses (sight, hearing, touch, and smell) to gain all the relevant information. For example, if you *see* cloudy urine, you *smell* it to check its odor.

Ask the following questions:

1. **How do my patient's data compare with accepted standards for normalcy for someone of this age, culture, disease process, and lifestyle?** If the person's data aren't within normal accepted standards, they are *abnormal* and considered a possible *sign* or *symptom* of a problem.
2. **Is my patient taking any medications that affect what would be considered normal?** Check action and side effects of all medications.
3. **How do my patient's current data compare with the previously collected data?** This question is especially helpful in situations where the patient has chronic signs and symptoms and you're trying to decide whether the signs and symptoms are getting worse.

For example, an asthmatic may always be slightly wheezy. However, if this same person is now wheezier than before, consider this increased wheeziness to be a sign of increasing problems.

Practice Exercises: Distinguishing Normal from Abnormal/Identifying Signs and Symptoms

Example responses are on pages 244 and 245.

1. Place an "S" next to the data below that either are signs or symptoms of a possible problem or signs or symptoms of a problem that's getting worse. Place an "O" if it's neither a sign nor a symptom. Place a question mark if you need more information to decide.
    a. Temperature of 99.6° F.
    b. Bilateral pulmonary rales.
    c. Someone tells you she rarely sleeps more than 3 hours at a time.
    d. Someone's nasogastric drainage has turned from brown to red.
    e. Someone's abdominal incision is slightly red around the sutures.
    f. A 2-year-old is inconsolable when his mother leaves the room.
    g. Someone with no health problems has developed ankle edema.
    h. Someone tells you they bathe every other week.
    i. Someone on kidney dialysis never urinates.
    j. Pulse of 54 per minute.
2. For each question mark you placed above, explain *what else* you'd want to know before you decided whether the information is abnormal (therefore a sign or a symptom).

5. MAKING INFERENCES (DRAWING VALID CONCLUSIONS)

Definition

Making deductions or forming opinions that follow logically by interpreting subjective and objective data. For example, note the data on the left below with the corresponding inferences on the right.

Data (Cues)	Corresponding Inference
Frowning	Seems worried
White blood cell count = 14,000	Probable infection
Deaf	Has communication problems

Why This Skill Promotes Critical Thinking

Your ability to interpret data and draw valid conclusions (make inferences) is essential to determining health status. If you draw some incorrect conclusions, your reasoning is likely to be flawed.

Making correct inferences helps you focus your assessment to look for *other information.* For example, if you infer that an elevated white blood cell count may indicate an infection, you know to look for signs and symptoms of infection.

Guidelines: How to Accomplish This Skill

The ability to make correct inferences requires problem-specific knowledge, knowledge of human behavior, and knowledge of cultural and spiritual influences. For example, to make the inference of *probable infection,* you need to know what a normal white blood cell count is *and* that an elevated white blood cell count is a sign of infection. Your knowledge of human behavior and spiritual and cultural influences is essential to making inferences about psychosocial data. For example, you may infer that someone's lack of eye contact indicates that he is mistrustful if you aren't aware that in his culture, lack of eye contact indicates respect.

It's important to remember the following rule.

▨ Rule
- Avoid making inferences based on only one cue (the more facts you have to support your inference, the more likely it is that your inference is correct).
- Once you make an inference, verify whether it's correct by gathering more information.

To avoid jumping to conclusions, begin your statements about inferences by saying, *I suspect this information indicates.* . . . Using this phrase reinforces that you to need to collect more data to decide if your suspicions are correct. Once you have enough evidence to support your inference you can begin to view it as *fact.*

Practice Exercises: Making Inferences (Drawing Valid Conclusions)

Example responses are on page 245.

Make an inference about each of the following data (begin your inference by writing, I suspect this information indicates. . .).

1. Temperature of 102° F. for 3 days.
2. A mother tells you she can't afford prenatal care.

3. A diabetic is 100 pounds overweight and says his blood sugar is always out of control, even though he watches his food intake and takes his insulin regularly.
4. A 5-year-old child whose mother told you he broke his leg falling down the stairs keeps looking at his mother before answering any of your questions.
5. A grandmother who usually is alert and active in her church presents with an unkempt appearance and seems a bit confused.

6. CLUSTERING RELATED CUES (DATA)

Definition

Grouping data in such a way that it helps you see relationships among the data. For example, you may have grouped the following cues together:

*   Two years old, temperature 100, pulse 144 per minute, rash all over trunk, recent measles exposure, never had measles, screaming that he wants his mother.

If you consider the relationship among the above data, you may suspect that the child's rapid pulse is related to his screaming rather than a sign of cardiac problems. If you consider all of the above data, you'll probably suspect these symptoms indicate the child may have measles.

Why This Skill Promotes Critical Thinking

Grouping information together applies the scientific principle of classifying information to enhance ability to see relationships between and among data. It helps you get a beginning picture of patterns of health or illness. A good way to remember the importance of clustering related data together is what I call "the puzzle analogy." When you put together a puzzle, you often begin by putting all the edges of the picture in one pile, all the pieces of a certain color in another pile, and so on. Putting the pieces in piles helps you begin to see patterns. The same principle applies to health assessment data, only in health care you cluster *signs and symptoms*.

Guidelines: How to Accomplish This Skill

1. How you cluster data depends on your purpose:
   - If you're trying to determine the status of medical problems or physiologic responses, cluster the data according to body systems (see Fig. 3–3, page 80).
   - If you're trying to determine the status of nursing problems, cluster the data according to a nursing model (e.g., see Box 3–5 or 3–6, pages 80 and 81.

Practice Exercises: Clustering Related Cues (Data)

Example responses are on page 245.

Read the following scenarios; then answer the questions that follow them.

Scenario One

The 16-year-old baby sitter next door calls and tells you that Jackson, the 7-year-old she's watching, was stung by a bee on the ear an hour ago. She tells you the ear is swollen and asks if you'll come and check him to decide whether he needs to go to the hospital. You go over and examine the child. He asks you if he might die "like the kid on *911* almost did." The baby sitter tells you she's afraid because she doesn't know where the mother is. You check the ear and find it red, swollen, and free of the stinger. When asked, Jackson tells you he was stung before but that wasn't as scary. Jackson has no rash and no wheezing. He asks if he could have a popsicle and watch TV. His pulse and respirations are normal.

a. Cluster the available information that will help you determine Jackson's physical health status.
b. Cluster the available information that will help you determine Jackson's human responses.
c. Cluster the available information that will help you determine the baby sitter's learning needs.

Scenario Two

It's 11 AM and you just admitted Mr. Nelson, a 41-year-old businessman who has acute abdominal pain. He's never been in the hospital and tells you he hates everything about hospitals. He's been vomiting for 2 days and unable to keep any food down. His abdomen is distended and he has no bowel sounds. He is scheduled to go to the operating room at 2 PM for emergency exploratory surgery. He's telling you he's worried because his brother died in the hospital after a car accident, when suddenly he doubles over and says, "Oh God, this is really getting worse!" You take his vital signs, and they are as follows: T 101 P 132 R 32 BP 140/80. These signs are the same as those taken an hour ago, except that before, his pulse was 104.

a. Cluster available information that will help you determine Mr. Nelson's physical status.

b. Cluster available information that will help you determine Mr. Nelson's human responses.

7. DISTINGUISHING RELEVANT FROM IRRELEVANT

Definition

Deciding what information is pertinent to understanding the situations at hand and what information is immaterial.

Why This Skill Promotes Critical Thinking

When faced with a lot of information, narrowing it down to *only the pertinent facts* prevents your brain from being cluttered with *unnecessary* facts. Deciding what's relevant is also an example of one of the principles of the scientific method: classifying or categorizing information into groups of related (relevant) information.

Guidelines: How to Accomplish This Skill

This skill is closely related to the previous skill, *clustering related cues*. However, we're looking at this skill in a little different way. In clustering data we simply put related information together. In this skill we look at the data we clustered together and decide what information is relevant *to a specific health concern*. You might say that you're now going to cluster the information in a different way. For example, you may have clustered *poor appetite* under nutrition and *productive cough* under respiratory system. You may decide that these two cues are relevant to deciding whether your patient has *pneumonia*. Keep in mind that organizing and reorganizing information promotes critical thinking because you see different relationships and patterns by doing this.

  Distinguishing relevant from irrelevant is especially difficult for novices. They tend to find themselves asking, How can I decide what's relevant if I don't know very much about the *problems* yet? Being able to decide what's relevant *does* depend on having problem-specific knowledge and experience. For instance, if you have a patient with a heart problem, you need to know the common causes and usual progression of heart problems to decide what information is relevant (e.g., if you know that *ankle edema* is an early sign of congestive heart failure, you recognize it as being a *relevant sign* to consider when determining cardiac status).

Here are some strategies that can help you determine what's relevant, even with limited knowledge:

1. List the abnormal data collected.
2. Then ask yourself, Could there be any connection between this (abnormal data) and that (abnormal data)?
3. As appropriate, ask the person or significant others, Do you think there's any relationship between this (abnormal data) and that (abnormal data)?
4. Data that might be connected to other data are likely to be relevant.
5. To decide specifically if a piece of information is relevant to a problem, compare the person's signs, symptoms, and risk factors with the signs, symptoms, and risk factors of the problem you suspect. For example, if the person has no support systems and you suspect *Ineffective Coping*, you'd consider no support systems as being relevant because lack of support systems is a risk factor for *Ineffective Coping*.

Practice Exercises: Distinguishing Relevant from Irrelevant

Example responses are on pages 245 and 246.

Consider the following scenarios; then answer the questions that follow them.

Scenario One

You're working in community health and are making a weekly visit to Mrs. Blondell, who is 80 years old and had a cerebrovascular accident (CVA) a month ago. Today you notice she seems to be increasingly confused: She knows where she is but forgets what day it is and doesn't seem to remember her daily routine.

You know that confusion in the elderly can be caused by any of the following: medications, infection, decreased oxygen to the brain, electrolyte imbalance, and brain pathology. You assess Mrs. Blondell and gather the data listed below. Consider each piece of the following information and decide its possible relevance to the problem of confusion: List whether you think it's relevant and why.

a. Recently started taking buspirone hydrochloride for anxiety
b. Temperature: 100° F. orally
c. History of a myocardial infarction 5 years ago

d. Seems dehydrated
e. Has no allergies
f. Regular diet

Scenario Two

You assess Mrs. Clark, a 32-year-old diabetic who is in for a routine visit. When you ask how the new diet is going, she breaks down into tears, saying, "I'm *never* going to be able to do this!"

Consider each piece of information below and decide its possible relevance to the problem with sticking to the diabetic diet: List whether you think it's relevant and why.

a. Diagnosed with diabetes 2 months ago
b. Vital signs within normal limits
c. Complains of constipation
d. Married with three school-age children
e. Loves to cook
f. Has always been 50 pounds overweight
g. Allergic to aspirin

8. RECOGNIZING INCONSISTENCIES

Definition

Realizing when there is conflicting information. For example, suppose you have someone who tells you he has no pain after chest surgery. However, he moves very little, guards his chest carefully, and barely breathes when you ask him to take a deep breath. The way this person is moving is *inconsistent* with his statements of being pain free.

Why This Skill Promotes Critical Thinking

Recognizing inconsistencies prompts you to investigate issues more closely. It sends up a red flag that tells you that you're going to have to probe more deeply to get the facts. It also helps you focus assessment to clarify the issues. For example, in the above case, you might say, "It seems to me that you aren't moving very well. I suspect you're having more pain than you admit. I want you to be comfortable, so that you move well and are able to take deep breaths to clear your lungs. Are you sure there isn't a particular spot that's causing you discomfort?"

Guidelines: How to Accomplish This Skill

One way to recognize inconsistencies is to compare what the patient states (subjective data) with what you observe (objective data). If what the person *states* isn't supported by what you *observe,* as in the preceding example, you've identified inconsistent information and need to investigate further.

Recognizing inconsistencies also requires a problem-specific knowledge. For example: Suppose your neighbor tells you, "I've been staying in bed because I strained my back. The right side is killing me." On further questioning, she says she also has a fever and cloudy urine. What would you suspect? If you're knowledgeable about how back injuries present, you'd recognize that the symptoms are *inconsistent* with a back injury and more consistent with a urinary tract infection.

To recognize these types of inconsistencies with limited knowledge:

1. Determine the signs and symptoms of the problem you suspect by looking up the problem in a reference (e.g., if you suspect pneumonia, look up the signs and symptoms of pneumonia in a textbook).
2. Compare the information in the reference with your patient's data. If your patient's signs and symptoms are *different* from those listed in the reference, you've identified inconsistencies and must investigate further: Assess the person more closely and consider other problems that the signs and symptoms might represent.

Practice Exercises: Recognizing Inconsistencies

Example responses are on page 246.

Read the following scenarios; then answer the questions that follow them.

Scenario One

You're interviewing Cathy in the prenatal clinic 2 weeks before delivery. You ask her how she feels about the baby coming. She tells you she's happy that she'll get to see the baby in only 2 weeks. When you ask her if she has any questions about the delivery, she tells you she's been going to birthing classes with her boyfriend and feels like she knows what to expect.

You review her records and notice that her first clinic visit was 2 weeks ago, when she came with her mother.

a. Identify inconsistencies in the above scenario.
b. Explain what you might do to clarify the inconsistencies you identified above.

Scenario Two

You're in the grocery store and a woman who appears to be about 20 years old comes up to you and says, "Please help me! I can't breathe, and my heart is racing. I think I'm having a heart attack!" You help her sit down, then take her pulse, and find it to be 100 per minute, regular, and strong; her respirations are 32 per minute. She tells you she has no pain but asks the store manager to call an ambulance. As you're waiting for the ambulance, she tells you this has happened to her several times before and that she has had an electrocardiogram, which showed normal cardiac function. Then she says, "But I *know* I'm having a heart attack! I'm so scared!"

• How consistent are this woman's signs, symptoms, and risk factors with those of a cardiac problem?

9. IDENTIFYING PATTERNS

Definition

Interpreting what patterns of function are suggested by the data you clustered together.

Why This Skill Promotes Critical Thinking

Identifying patterns helps you to form a *beginning picture* of the problems and also to recognize gaps in data collection. Once you recognize gaps in data collection, you can decide how to focus assessment to gain that missing information.

Here's an example of how identifying patterns helps you discover missing pieces of information. Suppose you clustered together the following cues:

• No bowel movement in 3 days
• Abdominal fullness
• States he's been "constipated off and on for the past month"

You may recognize that these cues represent a pattern of *Altered Bowel Elimination*. Having recognized this pattern, you know to focus your assessment to gain more information and decide *exactly* what the problem with bowel elimination is. For example: You ask, "What does *off and on* mean?" The person responds, "I get so constipated I have to take laxatives, and then I get diarrhea." This added information is likely to make you suspect that the bowel elimination problem is being caused in part by laxative abuse. You can then explore his knowledge of problems caused by laxative use.

Guidelines: How to Accomplish This Skill

Identifying patterns requires knowledge of *usual function* and *risk factors* for abnormal function. For example, to recognize *abnormal* coping patterns, you need to know *normal* coping patterns; to recognize potential (risk) for abnormal coping patterns, you need to know the *risk factors* for abnormal coping patterns (for example, social isolation, mental illness).
    To identify patterns:

1. Analyze the cues you clustered together and decide which of the following categories they represent:
    - **Normal pattern of function:** You identified *no* signs and symptoms.
    - **Potential (risk) for abnormal pattern of function:** You identified *risk* factors but no signs and symptoms. For example, if your patient has little fiber intake, minimal exercise, and takes frequent laxatives, he has a potential (risk) for *Altered Bowel Elimination,* even if today he had a normal bowel movement.
    - **Abnormal pattern of function:** You identified *signs and symptoms.* For example, your patient complains of constipation and hasn't had a bowel movement in 3 days.
2. Once you have a beginning idea of the patterns, ask, What *other* information might help me clarify my understanding of this pattern? Then collect that information.

Practice Exercises: Identifying Patterns

Example responses are on page 246.
    Consider the data listed for each letter *a* to *e* below. Then choose which one of the following patterns best describes the cluster of data and explain why.

- Potential (Risk) for Altered Bowel Elimination Pattern
- Potential (Risk) for Altered Sexual-Reproductive Pattern
- Probably Normal Sleep-Rest Pattern
- Altered Respiratory Function Pattern
- Probably Normal Coping Pattern

a. Bilateral rales; respirations increased to 34 per minute; coughing up thick, white mucus.

b. States, "I can cope with my illness, so long as I have help from my husband." Manages daily self-care; has husband cook all meals; passes the time by knitting blankets for the homeless.

c. Eats little roughage; just started taking codeine every 4 hours; drinks about 3 glasses of water daily; spends most of her time in bed; normal bowel function.

d. Works nights; sleeps 4 hours in the morning and 3 hours just before going to work at night.

e. Has just been diagnosed with genital herpes; single; worried about transmitting herpes to future sex partners and future children (during delivery).

10. IDENTIFYING MISSING INFORMATION

Definition

Recognizing gaps in data collection and searching for information to fill in the gaps.

Why This Skill Promotes Critical Thinking

Recognizing gaps in information and filling in those gaps prevent you from making one of the most common critical thinking errors: making judgments based on incomplete information. It also helps you clarify your understanding of the situations at hand.

Guidelines: How to Accomplish This Skill

1. One of the best ways to identify missing information is to analyze your written information and ask, What's missing here? When you

have all the information before you, your brain can more readily recognize what's missing than when going over the information mentally.

2. Other strategies for recognizing missing information include accomplishing all of the following critical thinking skills:
   - *Identifying assumptions*
   - *Checking accuracy and reliability of data*
   - *Clustering related cues*
   - *Recognizing inconsistencies*
   - *Identifying patterns*
   - *Evaluating and correcting thinking*

Practice Exercises: Identifying Missing Information

Example responses are on page 246.

Go back to the practice exercises for the previous skill, *identifying patterns*. For each pattern represented by the information listed in *a* to *e*, decide what information might be missing that could add to your understanding of the pattern.

11. PROMOTING HEALTH BY IDENTIFYING RISK FACTORS*

Definition

Improving health by early detection of factors that cause or put someone at risk for health problems.

Why This Skill Promotes Critical Thinking

Critical thinking is proactive. We don't wait for problems to appear to put a plan into action. By identifying risk factors, we think in a *disease prevention and health promotion mode* while the person is healthy.

---

*This skill deals with identifying risk factors *in healthy people*. The next skill deals with risk factors in the context of people with *existing health problems*.

Guidelines: How to Accomplish This Skill

1. Assess awareness of and motivation for identifying and managing risk factors. For example, determine whether they know what's required for adequate nutrition, rest, exercise, and spiritual and psychological well-being and whether they're willing to do what's needed. Not knowing about risk factors and not wanting to do something about them *are* risk factors.

2. Keep growth and development in mind. For example, a woman who is planning on becoming pregnant or *is* pregnant must consider risk factors for both herself and her baby.

3. Look for risk factors that are known to put people at risk for a variety of common problems. Some common examples:
   - Obesity, poor diet, high cholesterol, tobacco use, immobility, sedentary life, stressful life, poor sleeping habits, allergies, chronic illness, extremes of age (very young or old),low socioeconomic status, illiteracy, sun exposure, excessive use of medications, alcohol, or illicit drugs.

4. Also assess for:
   - Genetic, cultural, or biological factors (e.g., race, family history, and personal history predisposing one to health problems).
   - Behavioral factors (e.g., problems with anger management, attention deficit disorders).
   - Psychosocial/economic factors (e.g., lack of significant others, poverty)
   - Environmental factors (e.g., air quality).
   - Age-related factors (e.g., women after menopause are at risk for osteoporosis; infants are at risk for ear infection).
   - Sexual pattern factors (e.g., whether one is sexually active and with whom).
   - Safety-related factors (e.g., whether seat belts are worn, whether the home environment is safe for children).
   - Disease-related factors (e.g., someone with chronic lung disease is at risk for pneumonia; someone with diabetes is at risk for skin problems).
   - Treatment-related factors (e.g., complicated medication or treatment regimen).

■ **Want to Know More?** Find two excellent tables addressing *risk factors, related potential problems, and self-care strategies* and *screening procedures for health management behaviors across the life span* on pages 198–204 and 208–210 of Black, J., and Matassarin-Jacobs,

E. (1997). *Medical-Surgical Nursing* (5th ed.). Philadelphia: Saunders. **Also recommended:** (1) Health Seeking Behaviors (pp. 450–457) and Altered Health Maintenance (pp. 427–450). In L. Carpenito. (1997). *Nursing diagnosis: Application to clinical practice* (7th ed.). Philadelphia: Lippincott-Raven. (2) Department of Health and Human Services. Public Health Services. (1990). *Healthy people 2000: Promotion and disease prevention objectives* (DHHS Publication No. 91). Washington, DC: U.S. Government Printing Office.

Practice Exercises: Promoting Health by Identifying Risk Factors

Example responses are on page 247.

1. You assess a 25-year-old man and determine that he is healthy. What questions might you ask to identify risk factors for possible problems?
2. You assess a 72-year-old woman. You perform an assessment and find that she is healthy, but she does admit to being clumsy and tending to fall. In relation to normally encountered risk factors for a woman of this age, why should you be concerned about this?
3. You're at a barbecue talking casually with a 50-year-old man. He says, "You know I guess I'm getting to the age where I should be doing more to look after myself. How can I find out my risk factors?" What's your response?

12. DIAGNOSING ACTUAL AND POTENTIAL (RISK) PROBLEMS

Definition

Naming the problems that are present or may become present based on evidence from the heath assessment. This skill includes choosing a diagnostic label that best describes the problem and providing the evidence that leads you to believe the diagnosis is present.

Why This Skill Promotes Critical Thinking

In the context of the predict, prevent, and manage (PPM) approach to delivering health care, this skill is important for three reasons:

1. **Making definitive diagnoses (diagnosing actual and potential problems and their causes)** is essential to being able to deter-

mine *specific actions* designed to monitor, prevent, resolve, or control them.

2. **Predicting potential problems** also helps you:
   - Know what signs and symptoms to look for, and
   - Imagine scenarios that could happen (therefore allowing you to plan ahead)
3. **Providing the supporting evidence** that led you to conclude exactly what the actual and potential problems are helps you and others *evaluate thinking,* a skill that we'll address later. For example, consider the two problem statements below. Which one helps you better evaluate the thinking that led to the conclusion that there is a potential for violence?
   - *Potential for Violence*
   - *Potential for Violence related to a history of combative behavior and failure to attend anger management courses*

To grasp the importance of being able to accurately diagnose actual and potential problems, think about what can happen when you make a diagnostic error:

■   **Rule:** Diagnostic errors (missing problems or naming them incorrectly) can cause you to:
- Initiate actions that aggravate the problems or waste time.
- Omit essential actions required to prevent and manage the problems.
- Allow problems to go untreated.
- Influence others to believe the problems exist as described incorrectly.

Guidelines: How to Accomplish This Skill

The ability to identify and predict problems depends on knowledge and clinical expertise. Experts usually are able to identify problems much more quickly than novices because they've "seen it all before." They generate better hypotheses (they have better hunches about what the problems are), and they move through the steps of problem identification in a very dynamic way.[1]

If your knowledge and expertise are limited, you have an increased risk of making any one of the following mistakes.

- Overvaluing the probability of one diagnosis
- Not considering all the relevant data because of a narrow focus

- Failing to recognize personal biases or assumptions
- Making a diagnosis that's too general
- Overanalyzing ("analysis paralysis") and delaying taking action

Knowing that beginning nurses are at risk for the above mistakes helps them and more experienced nurses to *look for these types of errors* so that they can be corrected early.

The following guidelines are presented for identifying actual and potential (risk) problems:

Identifying Actual Problems

1. Verify that your information is correct and complete.
2. Avoid drawing conclusions or identifying problems based on only one cue. The more cues you have to support your conclusions, the more likely it is that your conclusions are valid.
3. Cluster abnormal data (signs and symptoms): Cluster according to body systems to identify medical problems and a nursing model to identify nursing problems.
4. Consider the signs and symptoms and ask yourself what information you could have missed.
5. Create a list of suspected problems that may be suggested by the signs and symptoms. Remember the following rule.

> ■ **Rule:** If you're not sure where to start when trying to create a suspected problem list, REPORT SIGNS AND SYMPTOMS immediately to expedite (hasten) problem identification and ensure patient safety. Even if you don't understand the problems, reporting signs and symptoms is a valuable and important step in expediting treatment.

6. After you complete your list of suspected problems, compare your patient's signs and symptoms with the signs and symptoms or defining characteristics of the problems you listed.
   - Some look at this phase as testing hypotheses (testing your hunches about what the problems may be).
7. Name the problems by choosing the diagnoses that *most closely resemble* your patient's signs and symptoms.
8. Determine *what's causing or contributing to the problems*
   - Always ask yourself whether it's possible that untreated (or inadequately treated) medical problems are causing the problems. If so, initiate a medical consultation immediately.

- Ask the person and significant others if they can identify factors that are contributing to the problems.
- Consider whether there are factors related to age, disease process, medications, or life changes that could be contributing to the problems.
- Look up the diagnoses you identified and check common related or causative factors; then assess your patient to determine whether he or she exhibits any of these factors.

9. As appropriate, use the mnemonic PRE (problem, related factors, evidence) and develop a problem statement that describes the:
   - Problem
   - Related factors (cause, risk factors)
   - Evidence that led you to conclude the problem exists

   Use *related to* to link the problem and its cause. For example:
   Pain related to left rib fracture as evidenced by statements of extreme tenderness in the left rib cage area.

Predicting Potential Problems

For nursing problems and diagnoses:
- Cluster data that indicate risk factors for problems. For example, you may cluster the following data: immobile, elderly, fragile skin.
- Name the potential (risk) problem by stating the problem and the risk factors, using *related to* to link the problem and risk factors. For example:
  Risk for Impaired Skin Integrity related to immobility and fragile skin.

For potential complications, consider:
- Medical problems, medications, and treatments present
- Whether invasive monitoring or diagnostic modalities were used recently
- What common potential complications are associated with the above. For example, if your patient just had a myocardial infarction (MI) and has an invasive monitoring device in place, determine common potential complications of MI (e.g., congestive heart failure, arrhythmias, pericarditis, MI extension, and cardiac arrest) and of the monitoring device (e.g., emboli)

Describe the potential complication by using the letters *PC,* followed by a colon.[2] For example:

PC: hemorrhage   or   *PC: increased intracranial pressure*

Practice Exercises: Diagnosing Actual and Potential (Risk) Problems

Example responses are on page 247.

Scenario One

You just admitted Nigel to the psychiatric unit. He is agitated but won't talk to anyone. You check previous records and note that he has a history of striking caregivers.

Write a diagnostic statement that best describes this potential problem by stating the problem and its related factors.

Scenario Two

Elaine is in the recovery room after having an emergency appendectomy under general anesthesia. She's very groggy and extremely nauseated.

Based on the above information, predict the potential complications Elaine might experience.

Scenario Three

You clustered together the following data: Mrs. Pue has just been told she has terminal cancer. She refuses to take her medications. She sleeps most of the time and says she doesn't want to talk to anyone. Mrs. Pue states her situation is hopeless and she's going to die so she'd rather not bother talking.

Based on the above information write a problem statement that best describes the problem using the PRE format.

Scenario Four

You're caring for a 41-year-old man who has four fractured ribs. What risk factors might you look for to determine whether he is at high risk for respiratory problems?

13. SETTING PRIORITIES

Definition

Differentiating between problems needing immediate attention and those requiring subsequent action; deciding what problems *must* be addressed on the plan of care.

Why This Skill Promotes Critical Thinking

Deciding what must be done first and what's most important helps you avoid an inefficient, possibly dangerous approach to problem solving. There are at least three major reasons why this skill is important:

1. Delays in treating some problems can cause severe consequences. For example, if you don't treat congestive heart failure *early*, it can progress to pulmonary edema.
2. By identifying relationships between problems and treating the ones that are contributing to *other* problems first, you avoid "quick fixes" and develop a safe, effective plan that's more likely to achieve long-term beneficial results. For example, if you treat pain with medication before determining its cause, you may resolve the pain but mask symptoms that require treatment.
3. If you give equal attention to *major* and *minor* problems, you may not be able to devote the time you need to resolving the problems that *must* be addressed to meet the overall expected outcomes.

Guidelines: How to Accomplish This Skill

Setting priorities happens in two phases:
1. Identify problems requiring immediate attention and initiate treatment as indicated (see Box 3–10, page 91).
2. After initiating essential early treatment, determine what problems *must* be addressed in the patient record to achieve the major outcomes of care.
   • Determine an overall expected outcome. For example, client will return home able to manage health care independently. (How to determine expected outcomes is addressed in the next skill. To help you complete this section, outcomes are provided for you.)

BOX 5–1	**Setting Priorities According to Maslow's Hierarchy of Human Needs**

No. 1 priorities: problems with survival needs (e.g., food, fluids, oxygen, elimination, warmth, physical comfort)

No. 2 priorities: problems with safety and security needs (e.g., risks of injury or infection, threats to feeling secure)

No. 3 priorities: problems with love and belonging (e.g., family problems, separation from loved ones)

No. 4 priorities: problems with self-esteem needs (e.g., need for privacy, respect, independence, and positive self-image)

No. 5 priorities: problems with self-actualization needs (e.g., need to grow and achieve outcomes)

Summarized from Maslow, A. (1970). *Motivation in personality.* New York: Harper & Row.

- Be sure you identify underlying causes of problems. Assign *management of causes* of problems a high priority (preventing, resolving, or controlling *causes* is crucial to preventing, resolving, or controlling the *problems*).
- List the problems; then determine whether there are relationships between the problems (consider whether one problem is contributing to another). Place a high priority on problems that contribute to other problems.
- Be sure nursing problems are given proper priority by using a method such as the one presented in Box 5–1.
- Determine which problems are addressed by facility standards, policies, procedures, or critical paths. For example, management of a fractured hip is likely to be addressed on a critical path (see page 257).
- Assign a high priority to recording a plan of care for the following problems: (1) those not covered by facility standard plans, protocols, or physician's orders; (2) those that may jeopardize achieving the major expected outcomes of the plan of care. These *must* be recorded.

Practice Exercises: Setting Priorities

Example responses are on page 247.

1. If the expected outcome is *will be discharged home by 7/28 able to manage colostomy care,* which of the following *must* be addressed on the plan of care?
   a. *Anxiety related to inability to return to work for 6 weeks*
   b. *Knowledge Deficit: Colostomy care*
   c. *Risk for Impaired Skin Integrity related to colostomy*
2. Read the following scenarios; then answer the questions that follow them.

Scenario One

Mr. Santos, a 64-year-old Guatemalan migrant worker, is admitted with a right calf thrombophlebitis. He is on bed rest, warm soaks, and anticoagulants. His knowledge of English is minimal. Today you try to teach him how to give himself anticoagulant injections. You have problems communicating, so you're thinking you should contact social services to get a translator to attend the teaching sessions. Mr. Santos is able to convey to you that his leg is still painful and that he's also been getting pains in his chest.

Based on the above information, what's your most *immediate* priority?

Scenario Two

You're looking after Neil, a 16-year-old football player who had surgery for a ruptured spleen 10 hours earlier. He is alert, his vital signs are stable, and his abdominal dressing is clean and dry. He has some incisional discomfort and hasn't been medicated for pain since surgery. He is also uncomfortable because he hasn't been able to void since surgery. He says, "I feel so lousy, I wish my mother could stay with me." When you offer to call her, he replies, "No, she's dying of cancer. I don't know what I'm going to do without her. Would you call my aunt?"

1. You've identified the following nursing concerns. Using Box 5–1 as a guide, decide how you would prioritize the needs/problems below: Place a "1" (for first priority), "2" (second priority), or "3" (third priority) in the appropriate blank.
   a. _____Wants his aunt to come in
   b. _____Hasn't voided
   c. _____Has incisional pain
2. Explain why you chose the order of priorities you listed above. (No example response provided.)

3. The expected outcome for Neil is, Will be discharged home by day 3 able to change dry sterile dressings. Neil demonstrates dressing changes the day after surgery and relates the importance of impeccable wound care. He is ambulatory and voiding well. Which of the following is *not required* to be addressed on the care plan and why?
   a. *Risk for infection related to incision*
   b. *Anticipatory grieving related to loss of his mother as evidenced by statements that mother has terminal cancer and he wishes she could be with him*
   c. *Knowledge deficit: dressing changes*

14. DETERMINING CLIENT-CENTERED EXPECTED OUTCOMES

Definition

Describing exactly what results will be observed *in the client* to show the anticipated benefits of the plan of care at a certain point in time.

Why This Skill Promotes Critical Thinking

Clearly describing *what beneficial results* will be observed *in the client* and at *what point* you expect to see them helps you:

- **Keep the focus on** *client responses,* the most important barometer for *measuring* how well the plan is working (you measure progress by comparing client responses with expected outcomes).
- **Determine priorities.** You need to know exactly what you're aiming to do before you can decide what's most important and what needs to be done first.
- **Get everyone motivated** (knowing the benefits and time frame for outcome achievement motivates clients and caregivers to initiate actions in a timely fashion).
- **Determine** *specific interventions* designed to achieve the outcomes. As the saying goes, If you don't know where you're going, it's hard to figure out how to get there.

Guidelines: How to Accomplish This Skill

Find out whether there are facility standard plans that address the expected outcomes for your patient's particular problems. These outcomes are often based on clinical evidence gathered over a period of time (therefore you have a good idea of *usual* expected results). If there are standard plans addressing outcomes, determine whether the outcomes are *appropriate* for your patient's particular situation (consider the outcomes in relation to things like age, presence of other problems, usual health state, home situation).

Even if your facility has already developed expected outcomes for certain problems, it's important that you know *principles* of identifying expected outcomes. Knowing the principles helps you know whether preestablished outcomes are appropriate for your specific patient situation. Knowing the principles is also crucial for developing outcomes for problems not addressed by preestablished plans.

Principles for Developing Expected Outcomes

1. Remember the following rule:

   ◼ **Rule:** *Expected outcomes* reflect the *benefits* expected to be observed *by others* after treatment is complete.

2. Expected outcomes may be written from a **problems** or **intervention** perspective.
   - Outcomes written for *problems* describe exactly what will be observed in the client to show that the problems are resolved (or controlled).
   - Outcomes written for *interventions* describe the *expected response* to the intervention.

   ◼ **Rule:** At a basic level, determining expected outcomes requires you to simply *reverse the problem* (state what happens when the person *doesn't* have the problem) or state the *desired response* to the intervention.

Example Problem	Corresponding Expected Outcome
Pain	Will relate being pain free or that pain level is managed to the point that it doesn't interfere with daily activities or sleep.
Example Intervention	
Nasogastric irrigation	Nasogastric tube will be patent.

3. Although some expected outcomes are written in a very abbreviated form, using only key words, remember the following rule.

■ **Rule:** To be clear and specific, expected outcome statements should have the following components:

Subject: *Who* is expected to achieve the outcome?
Verb: What will the person *do* (or what will be observed) to demonstrate outcome achievement?*
Condition: *Under what circumstances* will the person do it?
Performance Criteria: How *well* will the person do it?
Target Time: At *what point in time* will the person be able to do it?
Example: Tim will walk with a walker to the end of the hall by Friday.

4. Be sure you determine *overall* expected discharge outcome *first:* What will be observed *in this client* when care is terminated, and by when do you expect to observe it?
   Example: After three days the person will be able to demonstrate how to manage diabetes by monitoring his blood glucose and regulating his diet and insulin dosage.
5. Write outcomes for each problem that *must* be resolved or controlled to achieve the *overall* expected discharge outcome.
6. To determine daily outcomes, ask, *What will be observed in this client at the end of today after care has been delivered?*
   • Consider what will be the status of the *problems* and what will be the responses to the *interventions.*
7. Outcomes must be client centered: Make sure the *subject* of your outcome statement is the *client* or a *part of the client. Example: In-cision* will be free of signs of inflammation. (If the word *client* is implied, it's acceptable to omit the words *the client*).
8. Use verbs that are *observable and measurable* (actions you can clearly *see* or *hear*).
   • **Use verbs like** explain, describe, state, list, demonstrate, show, communicate, express, walk, gain, lose.
   • **Don't use verbs like** know, understand, appreciate, feel (these aren't measurable because no one can read someone else's mind to find out if they know, understand, appreciate, etc.).
9. If appropriate, use *as evidenced by* to describe exactly what you'll assess to determine if the outcome has been met. *Example:* The

---

*Sometimes it's not what the person will *do* but what will be *observed* in the client (for example, the client's skin will appear healthy and without signs of irritation or infection).

client will demonstrate knowledge of insulin management *as evidenced by* ability to state how insulin works, perform glucose monitoring, adjust insulin dose according to blood sugar level, and use sterile injection technique.

10. Share expected outcomes with key players (patient, significant others, other caregivers) to be sure that they're agreeable to those involved. Modify as needed.

■   **Want to Know More?** Find a comprehensive discussion of research on nursing outcomes in *Nursing Outcomes Classification (NOC)* by M. Johnson and M. Mass, St. Louis, MO: Mosby, 1997.

Practice Exercises: Determining Client-centered Expected Outcomes

Example responses are on page 248.

For each problem or intervention below, determine the most specific, client-centered outcome you can think of.

1. Risk For Impaired Skin Integrity related to age, obesity, and prolonged bed rest
2. Suction patient prn (as needed)
3. Powerlessness related to quadriplegia as evidenced by statements of, I have no choices
4. Irrigate Foley catheter every 4 hours
5. Endotracheal intubation
6. Activity Intolerance related to muscle weakness secondary to prolonged bed rest as evidenced by inability to walk the length of the hall without assistance

15. DETERMINING SPECIFIC INTERVENTIONS

Definition

Identifying specific nursing actions to prevent, control, or resolve problems and achieve outcomes efficiently by predicting responses, weighing risks and benefits, and tailoring actions to make them specific to the patient.

Why This Skill Promotes Critical Thinking

Identifying specific interventions designed to *increase* the likelihood of achieving the outcomes and *decrease* the likelihood of harm is crucial to developing a safe and efficient plan. Predicting the responses to interventions helps you be proactive: You can "test" interventions mentally before putting the plan into action. Having predicted the responses (both negative and positive) you can be more prepared. For example, you may think *this person may fall when I get him up, so I'd better have a second person there to help me.* Weighing risks against benefits helps you determine harmful interventions—you can decide whether your actions have a greater likelihood of causing harm than good. For example, in the previous case, you may decide not to get the person out of bed at all if you don't have a second person there to help you.

Describing very specific interventions increases the likelihood that the actions will be carried out as specified. Notice how *b* clearly describes the intervention as compared with *a.*

    a. Monitor breath sounds and help with coughing and deep breathing
    b. Monitor breath sounds and splint front left lower ribs while helping with coughing and deep breathing every 4 hours during waking hours

Guidelines: How to Accomplish This Skill

Even if your facility has already identified standard interventions for certain problems, it's important that you know *principles* of identifying interventions. Knowing the principles helps you decide whether preestablished interventions are appropriate for your specific patient situation. It's also crucial for identifying interventions for problems not addressed by preestablished plans.

Principles for Determining Interventions

    1. Remember the following rule:

       ■ **Rule:** To determine specific nursing interventions, consider *both* the problems and the expected outcomes.
       • Consider each problem and ask, What can be done about the *problem,* and what can be done about the problem's *cause or risk factors*?

• Consider the outcomes and ask, How can we *tailor the interventions* to achieve these specific outcomes?

2. Using the mnemonic **MPCR** (**M**onitor, **P**revent, **C**ontrol, **R**esolve), determine *specific* actions that will:
   • Monitor, prevent, resolve, or control the *cause* (risk factors) of the problems.
   • Monitor, prevent, resolve, or control the *problems*.
3. Decide whether you need to make the interventions more specific, based on expected outcomes.
   Example: You may have identified the intervention of increase fluid intake. An outcome for this patient states, will drink at least 2500 cc per day. To make the intervention specific for the outcome, you'd write something like, increase fluid intake during day shift to 1000 cc, during evening shift to 1000, and at night to 500 cc.
4. Include patients and significant others in tailoring interventions as much as possible. They are the ones who know themselves best.
5. Predict outcomes to your interventions (patient responses) and determine any risk of harm.
6. Fine-tune the interventions to include ways of increasing the likelihood of beneficial responses and decreasing the risk of harm.
7. Remember the words *see, do, teach, record.* Consider what you'd *see* (assess), what you'd *do*, what you'd *teach*, and what you'd *record*. *Example:*
   • **See (assess).** Assess ability to walk with walker in the room before allowing him to go out in the hall alone.
   • **Do.** Have him walk the length of the hall three times a day.
   • **Teach.** Reinforce that sticking to the plan will increase muscle strength and reduce fatigue.
   • **Record.** Record pulse and blood pressure before and after walking at least once a day.
   You may not always have to address all of the above, but you should consider whether you need to address each one.

◼ **Want to Know More?** Find a comprehensive discussion of research on nursing interventions impacting on patient care in *Nursing Intervention Classification (NIC)* (2nd ed.) by J. McCloskey and G. Bulechek, St. Louis, MO: Mosby-Year Book, 1996.

Practice Exercises: Determining Specific Interventions

Example responses are on page 248.

1. Determine specific interventions for each of the following problems.

Problems	Corresponding Expected Outcomes
a. Risk for Fluid Volume Deficit related to diarrhea and insufficient fluid intake.	Will maintain adequate hydration as evidenced by drinking at least 4 quarts per day
b. Anxiety related to insufficient knowledge of hospital procedures.	After being fully informed about hospital procedures, will express that anxiety is reduced.
c. Chronic Pain related to arthritic joints as evidenced by statements of suffering from arthritic pain in knees and hands for the past 20 years.	After application of heat and assistance with range of motion will express that knee pain is manageable.

2. Consider the following scenario; then respond to the questions that follow.

Scenario

You make a home visit to the Supopoffs, Russian immigrants who live in the suburbs in a church-sponsored home. The family has three children, aged 5, 7, and 10. The house they live in is adjacent to a tall grassy area, which is full of deer ticks. Mrs. Supopoff is upset because she keeps finding deer ticks on the children, and she knows Lyme's disease comes from deer tick bites. Even though she's told the children not to go into the grassy area, she suspects they disregard her instructions when playing. Mrs. Supopoff is considering punishing the children when she finds a tick on them, hoping this will make them more careful.

You look up Lyme's disease and learn that the best treatment For Lyme's is *prevention* of tick bites.

You identify the following problem and expected outcome:

Problem: Risk for Infection related to tick bites.
Expected outcome: The children will have a decreased risk of getting tick bites and infection as evidenced by wearing insect repellent when outside, avoidance of tall grass areas, and monitoring themselves and each other for ticks.

a. Consider the risks and benefits of the following actions:
   (1) What might happen if the children are punished when a tick was found on them?
   (2) What might happen if you reward the children for finding ticks?

b. What interventions might safely motivate the children to participate in spotting ticks?
c. Write specific interventions to achieve the above expected outcome.

16. EVALUATING AND CORRECTING THINKING

Definition

Looking for flaws in thinking, determining how well critical thinking skills were accomplished, and making necessary corrections.

Why This Skill Promotes Critical Thinking

Critical thinking is reflective, proactive, purposeful thinking that strives for accuracy and reliability. By forming the habit of constantly reflecting on and evaluating your thinking, asking yourself questions like, Am I clear about what's going on here? What am I missing? How can I be more sure that I'm using sound reasoning? Am I holding myself to high standards? and Should I be thinking of some creative approaches here? you can significantly improve the outcomes of your thinking.

Guidelines: How to Accomplish This Skill

As discussed in previous skills, evaluating and correcting thinking is an *ongoing* process. Box 5–2 provides the types of questions you should be asking at various points in the nursing process to evaluate and correct thinking.

There are no practice exercises for this skill, as opportunities for evaluating and correcting thinking have been provided throughout the other skills.

17. DETERMINING A COMPREHENSIVE PLAN/EVALUATING AND UPDATING THE PLAN

Definition

Ensuring that all major problems, outcomes, and interventions are recorded and evaluated in the patient's permanent record; keeping the plan up to date.

BOX 5-2	**Example Questions Asked to Evaluate and Correct Thinking at Various Stages of the Nursing Process**

1. **Assessment**
   - What assumptions could I have missed?
   - How complete is data collection?
   - How sure am I of the accuracy and reliability of the data?
   - How well do I understand my patient's perceptions?
   - How sure am I of the conclusions I've drawn (inferences I've made)?
   - Have I considered what data I need from both a nursing and medical perspective?
2. **Diagnosis**
   - How well does the evidence support that the problems I've identified are correct?
   - Have I missed any other problems that could be indicated by the evidence?
   - Am I clear about the underlying causes?
   - How clearly and specifically are the problems stated?
   - Am I clear about the definitive diagnoses here?
   - Have I identified both nursing problems and problems requiring a multidisciplinary approach?
   - Were client strengths and resources identified?
3. **Planning**
   - What immediate priorities could have been missed? Did I remember to include the patient and significant others in setting priorities?
   - Have I missed any problems that must be addressed on the plan of care?
   - How well do the outcomes reflect the benefits I expect to see?
   - Are the outcomes realistic, clear, and client centered?
   - Did I consider both the problems and the outcomes when identifying interventions?
   - Did I consider client preferences when developing the plan, and did I take advantage of client strengths and resources?
4. **Implementation**
   - Are the problems still the same?
   - Am I missing any new problems?
   - Am I keeping the focus on *client responses*?
   - Should I be doing anything differently? Are the interventions still appropriate?
5. **Evaluation**
   - How accurately and completely have I completed each of the previous steps?
   - What could I be doing differently/better?

Why This Skill Promotes Critical Thinking

Developing a comprehensive plan and ensuring that the major care plan components are recorded:

- Forces you to think about the *most important* aspects of giving care.
- Provides data for evaluation, research, legal, and insurance purposes.
- Promotes communication between caregivers (therefore improving thinking of the health care team).

Continuously thinking about how the plan is working and what changes must be made is essential to reaching outcomes efficiently.

Guidelines: How to Accomplish This Skill

1. Being able to determine a comprehensive plan requires all of the skills listed in this section and knowing the *purpose* and *components* of the recorded plan (see Box 5-3).
2. Identify the major problems and interventions yourself. Then:
   - Check the patient record to see whether the problems and interventions are addressed by preestablished plans, policies, or doctor's orders. For example, check whether policies, standard plans, or critical paths address care management of the problems you identify.

BOX 5-3   **Purpose and Components of the Recorded Plan of Care**

Purpose of Recorded Plan
- Promotes communication between caregivers
- Directs care, interventions, and documentation
- Creates a record that can later be used for evaluation, research, legal and insurance purposes

Components of Recorded Plan
- Expected outcomes
- Actual and potential problems that must be addressed to achieve the major outcomes of care
- Specific interventions designed to control or resolve the problems and achieve the outcomes
- Evaluation statements (progress notes)

- Compare your patient's situation with the interventions on pre-established plans. Modify or add interventions if needed.
3. To evaluate and update the plan, compare what's *supposed* to happen (or what you're supposed to find) as described in the standard plan with what you *actually* find when you assess the patient.
    - Determine progress toward expected outcomes for major problems. For example, if the expected outcome states *will be free of signs of infection around wound incision,* assess the incision for signs of infection (e.g., redness, drainage, heat, and tenderness).
    - Monitor status of problems closely; watch closely for new risk factors or problems. If risk factors or problems change, be sure the plan of care reflects this.
    - Monitor outcomes of interventions after each intervention. If you aren't seeing the expected results, start thinking about what you could change to improve the results.
    - Modify interventions as needed, changing the record as needed.
4. Remember the following rule.

■ **Rule: An essential daily nursing responsibility is looking for care variances and taking appropriate action.** A care variance is when a patient hasn't achieved activities or outcomes by the time frame noted on a critical path. Identifying a care variance should trigger you to think, What additional assessment do we need to do to determine whether this delay is justified? and What could we do to improve this person's likelihood of achieving the outcome? Think in terms of, *What resources and multidisciplinary approaches might help?*

Practice Exercises: Determining a Comprehensive Plan/Evaluating and Updating the Plan

Example responses are on pages 248 and 249.

1. Consider each of the expected outcomes and corresponding patient data and decide whether the outcome has been achieved, partially achieved, or not achieved.
    a. **Expected outcome:** Will be ready for discharge by day 3 after surgery as evidenced by ability to relate how to manage wound packing. **Patient data:** Doesn't feel managing wound packing should be his concern and feels he's incapable of doing so.
    b. **Expected outcome:** Will drink at least 4 quarts of fluid as evidenced by keeping a written record of fluid intake. **Patient data:** Record indicates 5 quarts of fluid intake daily.

      c. **Expected outcome:** The baby will be discharged home with parents able to perform CPR. **Parent's data:** Father demonstrates CPR well. Mother has trouble establishing airway.

2. Develop a comprehensive plan, identifying two priority diagnoses for the following scenario. Include an overall expected discharge outcome, outcomes for each diagnosis, and specific interventions.

> ### Scenario
>
> It's Monday. You admit Mrs. Kooney, who has just suffered anaphylactic shock after a bee sting. Mrs. Kooney is expected to be discharged by Wednesday June 29th. The doctor gives Mrs. Kooney an emergency epinephrine injection kit and tells her, "The nurse will teach you how to use it." Mrs. Kooney still has hives all over her body and says her itching feet are driving her crazy. You find that placing her feet in cool water every so often really helps her discomfort. She is still slightly wheezy from the bee sting reaction.
>
> When you ask her about using the injection kit, she replies "No way!" Her husband, who is retired, says, "I'll be glad to learn." It's decided that it's satisfactory to discharge Mrs. Kooney on June 29th, so long as her husband can demonstrate how to manage giving the epinephrine in an emergency.

3. Suppose you're using the critical path on page 257. Today is your patient's third postoperative day. The only significant data you find is that your patient is very confused. You compare this data with what's supposed to happen on the third postoperative day (second column on the path). What should you do and why?
4. Suppose you're reviewing someone's chart to determine if a comprehensive plan of care is present. What four care plan components will you be looking for?
5. Get an actual patient chart. Determine whether the four components of the plan of care are recorded (no response for this one).

CRITICAL MOMENTS

How Do You Know Whether to Trust an Expert?

If a little knowledge is dangerous, there are a lot of dangerous people walking around out there. Don't just assume others know more than you do, even if they sound knowledgeable: Ask questions, seek clarification, and think independently (e.g., Ask, Where might I find a reference to add to my knowledge of this?).

Footnotes/References

[1]Norman, G. (1988). Problem-solving skills, solving problems, and problem-based learning. *Medical Education, 22,* 279.

[2]Carpenito, L. (1997). *Nursing diagnosis: Application to clinical practice* (7th ed.). Philadelphia: Lippincott.

See comprehensive bibliography beginning on page 280.

6

Applied Critical Thinking: Mastering Common Workplace Skills

This chapter at a glance . . .

Read the Learning Outcomes listed at the beginning of each skill in this section. If you can readily achieve them, skip that particular skill. If you can achieve them all, skip this chapter.

HOW TO BEST USE THIS CHAPTER

This section is designed for group learning. To complete most critical thinking exercises, you need at least one other person. The best way to master the skills is to plan a seminar for each skill to promote in-depth discussion and thought. As part of the seminar requirements, each participant should read at least two up-to-date articles on the topic. References used for the content on each skill are provided at the end of the particular skill section.

ABSTRACT

This chapter provides strategies for mastering abilities related to the SCANS workplace skills (see Box 1-1, page 5). Organized alphabetically, each skill is presented in the following format: (1) Name of the Skill, (2) Definition of the Skill, (3) Learning Outcomes, (4) Thinking Critically about the Skill, (5) Strategies for Mastering the Skill, and (6) Critical Thinking Exercises.

1. ADAPTING TO AND FACILITATING CHANGE

Definition

Knowing how to function and grow when faced with change.

Learning Outcomes

After you study this information and complete the accompanying exercises you should be able to:

- Explain your own reaction when faced with change.
- Identify strategies that can help you adapt to change.
- Describe how to facilitate change in others.

Thinking Critically about Change

Even if you're on the right track, you still get hit by the train if you don't keep moving. I can't think of a saying that describes the need for change better than this one. Thriving in this rapidly changing world depends on your ability to deal effectively with responses to change (both your own and those of others). Knowing how to help yourself and others adapt to change reduces stress and maximizes productivity.

Strategies for Adapting to and Facilitating Change

Adapting to change:
1. Suspend judgment; fairly explore reasons for the required change.
2. Curb the tendency to be influenced by the natural desire to keep the status quo because it's easy and comfortable.

3. Make sure you understand why the change is being made and how you feel about it. If you can get something out of the change, it will help you accept it.

4. Identify barriers to making the change and find ways to deal with them. For example, if you have to start using new equipment, making yourself a "cheat sheet" can help you remember key information.

5. Ask for help. If you express the problems you're having, others may be able to help and you may also identify common concerns that are bothering everyone.

6. Don't be surprised if you go through the following natural sequence of events commonly associated with adapting to change:

   - **Losing focus:** Expect some confusion, disorientation, and forgetfulness at first. You may be unsure about boundaries and responsibilities. Ask for clarification, keep notes, and use to-do lists.

   - **Denial:** You may want to minimize or deny the effect the change has on you. However, connecting with and dealing with your feelings will help you move forward. Acknowledge how you feel about what you lose and gain by making the change.

   - **Anger/Depression:** Don't be surprised if you feel angry, discouraged, or frustrated.
     - Vent your anger in a safe place. Be careful with *whom, how, and where* you ventilate. Your words can come back to haunt you. Find someone who'll listen empathetically without being affected by your feelings (e.g., someone who has gone through the change you're experiencing, not someone who also is struggling and who may be pulled down by your negativity).
     - Use stress management strategies (e.g., exercise helps diffuse anger and frustration).
     - Keep away from negative people; their thoughts might influence you negatively.

   - **Acceptance:** Stay focused on what you'll gain from making the change. Be patient with yourself, let go of the past, and take it one step at a time. Make a conscious effort to think critically and not emotionally.

   - **Moving forward:** Seek opportunities to use the new skills and procedures you learned. Celebrate small successes, recognizing how far you've come and what you've learned along the way. Share your experience with those who may not have come as far as you have.

7. Remember to represent your organization positively in public, even if you don't feel that way at the moment.

Facilitating change in others

1. Imagine how the change will impact on those involved. Be clear about the positives and negatives from *their* perspective.
2. Clearly articulate both the changes required and the benefits of making the change.
3. Clarify changes in roles and responsibilities.
4. Get the backing of formal and informal group leaders and try to win them toward the change (they can help or hurt a lot).
5. Allow people to explore how the change will affect their daily lives. Encourage their involvement in finding ways to make the change easier.
6. Convey an understanding of negative feelings and extra work associated with having to make a change. Provide necessary resources and support (e.g., technical and decision support) until the change has been fully implemented
7. Ask for ownership of responsibility for change (both parties own some of the work).
8. Involving key players, identify barriers to making the change and find ways to deal with them. For example, if the staff is expected to take time to practice using a new computer system, provide extra personnel to do ordinary chores.
9. Be clear about time lines: Key players must know exactly what change is expected to occur and by when.
10. Be patient. Going through the stages of adapting to change takes time.

OTHER PERSPECTIVES

Don't Kid Yourself

"There's an illusion we can manage change by controlling the world around us."

—Mohandas Ghandi

CRITICAL MOMENT

Transform Rather Than Conform

When facilitating change, aim to *transform* rather than *conform*. Inspire, show benefits, encourage, and support. When people are transformed, they change because they want to.

Critical Thinking Exercises

In a group or in a journal entry:

1. Share your best and worst experiences with adapting to change and what factors made it your best and worst experiences.
2. Describe a personal or work change that you experienced that wasn't of your choice (e.g., moving, changing job description).
   - Think about how you felt at the time and the effect it had on your ability to make the change.
   - Identify some things you could have done to make the change easier.
3. Share a time you tried to help someone else change.
   - How successful were you?
   - What, if anything, would you do differently?
4. Study Box 6–1 (Four Ways We Change). Explain why paradigm change facilitates critical thinking.

BOX 6–1	**Four Ways We Change***

Four Ways We Change

1. Pendulum change: I was wrong before, but now I'm right.
2. Change by exception: I'm right, except for . . . .
3. Incremental change: I was *almost* right before, but *now* I'm right.
4. Paradigm change: What I knew before was *partially* right. What I know now is more right but only part of what I'll know tomorrow.

Paradigm Change Is Transformational

Paradigm change combines what's useful about *old ways* with what's useful about *new ways* and keeps us open to looking for *even better* ways.
We realize:
- Our previous views were only part of the picture.
- What we now know is only part of what we'll know later.
- Change is no longer threatening: It enlarges and enriches.
- The unknown can then be friendly and interesting.
- Each insight smooths the road, making the change process easier.

---

*Adapted and summarized from Ferguson, M. (1980). *Aquarian conspiracy: Personal and social transformation in our time.* New York: G. P. Putnam's Sons.

5. Explain the difference between change that transforms and change that conforms.
6. Determine whether you can achieve the Learning Outcomes at the beginning of this skill.

References

Ferguson, M. (1980). *Aquarian conspiracy: Personal and social transformation in our time.* New York: G. P. Putnam's Sons.

Giblin, C. (1996). *Dealing with change—creating a personal plan.* King of Prussia, PA: Organization Design and Development Inc.

Glaser, R., Glaser, C. (1995). *Building a winning team.* King of Prussia, PA: Organization Design and Development Inc.

Glaser, R., Glaser, C. (1995). *Team effectiveness profile.* King of Prussia, PA: Organization Design and Development Inc.

Grindel, C., Bayley, E., Kingston, M., et al. (1997). Nurses preparing for change: Their needs and concerns. *MEDSURG Nursing, 6*(5), 278–286.

Lancaster, J. (1999). *Nursing issues in leading and managing change.* St. Louis: Mosby.

Libove, L. (1996). *Leading change at every level.* King of Prussia, PA: Organization Design and Development Inc.

Manion, J. (1995). Understanding the seven stages of change. *American Journal of Nursing, 95*(4), 41–43.

2. COMMUNICATING BAD NEWS

Definition

Knowing how to convey honesty, empathy, and responsibility when giving someone information that will have a negative impact on them.

Learning Outcomes

After you study this information and complete the accompanying exercises you should be able to:

- Explain what can happen when you avoid giving bad news.
- Identify strategies to minimize the impact of bad news.
- Determine how you can reduce your stress when faced with giving bad news.

Thinking Critically about Bad News

No one likes having to be the messenger with bad news. All too often people who have bad news tend to avoid this unpleasant chore altogether, making things only worse. When you communicate bad news at an appropriate time, in an appropriate place, and with honesty, empathy, and responsibility, you can soften the blow by minimizing the common feelings of anger, disappointment, and betrayal.

How you handle giving bad news can make the difference between escalating an already difficult situation and building positive relationships in spite of adversity. Using the following strategies can help reduce your stress and give you more energy to focus on achieving a positive outcome (building a positive relationship in spite of adversity).

Strategies for Communicating Bad News

Steps	Example
1. Give the bad news in a timely way. Offer an apology and don't try to obscure the situation.	I'm sorry to tell you we won't be able to do your x-ray today.
2. Showing concern, explain what happened and why.	Somehow you were scheduled in our book for next week, but your appointment card says today. I'm not sure how this happened, but I'm going to find out.
3. Present alternative solutions and give pros and cons of each.	I could schedule the x-ray for later today, but we get better pictures if you fast for 12 hours before the x-ray. I realize you'd have to go home and come back and that you'd like to get it over with. I think it's worth waiting to be sure we get a good quality x-ray.
4. Recommend a course of action. Include: • How the plan addresses the problem. • How the plan addresses hardships resulting from what happened.	I think the best solution is to schedule the x-ray as soon as possible. Since you've already had enough problems, I'll do my best to schedule you whenever it's convenient for you. I'll also find out who made this mistake and see what we can do to prevent this from happening again.
5. Reaffirm your goals and vision for the future. Include: • Key points that give confidence to those involved. • Time frame for expected results.	We're here to serve you the best way we can. Soon we'll have a system that allows you to confirm an appointment over the phone. We hope to have the system in place by May. Everyone will be encouraged to call and confirm their appointments when they get home.

Steps	Example
6. Follow up to see if results were satisfactory.	I'll be sending your name to our community relations department. They will be calling you to see if everything was resolved to your satisfaction. Please feel free to call and discuss anything you'd like with them as well. We want you to feel satisfied with your experience with us.

Related Skills: Dealing with Complaints Constructively (page 195).

Critical Thinking Exercises

Instructions: In a group, in a personal journal, or both:

1. Describe:
   - Your best and worst experiences with how someone gave you bad news.
   - The emotions you feel when giving bad news.
   - How people you know have responded to bad news situations and why you think they responded that way.
2. Imagine you and five classmates or colleagues are responsible for making a presentation. The night before the presentation, your computer crashes and you lose your part of the presentation. How will you tell the group this?
3. On a computer that has Microsoft Powerpoint software, write a letter communicating imaginary bad news using the "Communicating Bad News" wizard.
4. Determine whether you can achieve the Learning Outcomes at the beginning of this skill.

References

Paulson, T. (1991). *They shoot managers, don't they?* Berkeley, CA: Ten Speed Press.

Rager, P. (1998). Emotional intelligence and the management edge. *Nursing Spectrum (FL ED), 8*(3), 3.

Weisinger, H. (1998). *Emotional intelligence at work.* San Francisco, CA: Jossey-Bass.

Weisinger, H., Lobsenz, N., (1983). *Nobody's perfect.* New York: Warner Books.

3. DEALING WITH COMPLAINTS CONSTRUCTIVELY

Definition

Using complaints as an opportunity to improve customer satisfaction.

Learning Outcomes

After you study this information and complete the accompanying exercises you should be able to:

- Explain the value of complaints.
- Deal with complaints with more competence.
- Express more confidence about dealing with complaints.

Thinking Critically about Complaints

Just thinking about dealing with complaints makes most of us squirm. However, if we recognize that complaints are useful, maybe we can change our attitude and greet this challenge in more positive ways. Think about the value of complaints:

Complaints are valuable. They help you:
- Correct problems before they become worse or happen to someone else.
- Identify trends in unmet needs of consumers.
- Find out about complaints before people start complaining to others.

Like all businesses, health care organizations thrive when consumers are happy. Satisfied consumers tell others about their experience and return as needed. The opposite is also true: If your consumers are unhappy, they tell others and they take their business elsewhere.

When someone complains, take time to listen and do something about it.

Strategies for Dealing with Complaints

1. **Start off on the right foot.** Don't take things personally. Assume there's a very good reason for the complaints (although these reasons may be unclear at first).

2. **Take a deep breath and remain calm** in the face of anger. People requiring health care often have extenuating circumstances that cause them to have a "short fuse." Some examples:
   - Previous bad experience with health care providers or treatment plans.
   - Effects of illness or disability on self, family, and work.
   - Problems of being in limbo (the patient may not be responding as quickly or favorably as expected).
   - Family reaction to illness or disability.
3. **Listen actively** to figure out what the person really values and needs.
   - Give the person your full attention.
   - Repeat what you hear to be sure that you're clear on the issues.
   - Aim to give them what they need or value if at all possible (this requires that you get a clear understanding from your boss about what rules you can bend or break to immediately resolve issues).
   - If you come in late to the situation, remain quiet, *listen*, and ask to verify your understanding of the problem.
4. **Focus on the issues** and try to learn from them.
5. **Swallow your pride,** offer an apology, and avoid weak excuses (we're short staffed; nobody's perfect). You'll move more quickly to a solution.
6. **Take some immediate step** to resolve the problem. Explain what you're going to do and let them feel like they're winning in some way.
7. **Involve the person** in problem solving (ask for solutions).
8. **Keep the person informed** (e.g., I promise to let you know the minute I know more about this).
9. **Report and record special needs.** Let your supervisor know about all major complaints or incidents.
10. **Follow up** to see if solutions are working.
11. **If anger explodes:**
    - Keep your own anger in check.
    - Don't defend yourself. Listen completely; focus keenly on what is being said.
    - Keep in mind that some people cope in ways you consider negative (abrasive, manipulative).
    - Think about whether having your manager come and talk with the person would help.

Related Skills: Communicating Bad News, Managing Conflicts Constructively, Giving and Taking Feedback, Developing Partnerships.

Critical Thinking Exercises

In a group or in a journal entry:

1. Address the feelings associated with making complaints (e.g., anger, guilt, frustration).
2. Give an example of a time when you thought about complaining but decided it just wasn't worth it. How did this make you feel, and who do you think lost in this situation?
3. Describe your best and worst experience with making a complaint.
4. Explain how you usually deal with complaints; then think of some ways you could improve your response.
5. Summarize and discuss the following article: Wolf, Z., Brennan, R., Ferchau, L., Magee, M., et al. (1997). Creating and implementing guidelines on caring for difficult patients: A research utilization project. *MEDSURG NURSING, 6*(3), 137–147.
6. Determine whether you can achieve the learning outcomes at the beginning of this skill.

References

Feuer, L. (1997). The customer from hell: Solutions and strategies (unpublished handouts). Medical Case Management Convention. September 30, Nashville, Tennessee.

Paulson, T. (1991). *They shoot managers, don't they?* Berkeley, CA: Ten Speed Press.

Rager, P. (1998). Emotional intelligence and the management edge. *Nursing Spectrum (FL ED), 8*(3), 3.

Russo, E. (1996). *Putting the customer first: Steps for building lasting relationships.* King of Prussia, PA: Organization Design and Development.

Weisinger, H. (1998). *Emotional intelligence at work.* San Francisco, CA: Jossey-Bass.

Wolf, Z., Brennan, R., Ferchau, L., Magee, M., et al. (1997). Creating and implementing guidelines on caring for difficult patients: A research utilization project. *MEDSURG NURSING, 6*(3), 137–147.

4. DEVELOPING EMPOWERED PARTNERSHIPS

Definition

Building mutually beneficial relationships based on the belief that people have the right and responsibility to make their own choices and grow in their own way.

Learning Outcomes

After you study this information and complete the accompanying exercises you should be able to:

- Compare and contrast a Parental Model* and an Empowered Partnership Model.
- Explain the benefits of empowered partnerships.
- Begin to build empowered partnerships.

Thinking Critically about Empowered Partnerships

Developing empowered partnerships with peers, colleagues, and patients requires a shift in thinking from a Parental Model (*I'll take care of you*) to an Empowered Partnership Model (*It's your life. You have rights and responsibilities as well as I do. I want to learn from my experience with you*).

The *I'll take care of you* way of doing things promotes dependency, is inefficient, and reduces growth and self-esteem. In contrast, the *I'll help you learn to take care of yourself* way of doing things promotes growth and self-esteem and gets results in a timely manner. To understand these two models, look at Table 6–1.

Many nurses with excellent intentions still function in a parental manner. They haven't made the shift in thinking to an empowered partnership that we know is so important to achieving quality outcomes. As nurses, we must encourage and empower peers, coworkers, patients, and families to take as much responsibility as possible for managing their own lives.

Strategies for Developing Empowered Partnerships

1. **Be sure you can explain the concept of an empowered partnership.**
   - An empowered partnership is a relationship in which the power between two people or groups is roughly balanced.[†] Although you can't completely balance power in all relationships, the aim of an empowered partnership is to balance the power as much as possible.

---

*Some people call this a Paternal Model. "Parental" is used to avoid sexism.

†Block, P. (1996). *Stewardship: Choosing service over self-interest.* San Francisco, CA: Berrett-Koehler, p. 28.

TABLE 6–1	**Phrases Exemplifying Two Relationship Models**

PHRASES EXEMPLIFYING PARENTAL MODEL	PHRASES EXEMPLIFYING EMPOWERED PARTNERSHIP
<ul><li>I want to look after you.</li><li>I know what's best for you.</li><li>You should do as I say.</li><li>I'm responsible for you.</li></ul>	<ul><li>How can I empower you to be able to be independent?</li><li>You know yourself best. Tell me what you'd like to see happen, what's most important to you.</li><li>I want you to be able to make informed choices.</li><li>We share a common purpose and we're both responsible for what happens.</li></ul>

Examples of Empowered Partnerships

Nurse-patient/client	Staff nurse–nurse manager
Teacher-student	Nurse-pharmacist
Nurse–unlicensed workers	Nurse-employer
Nurse-nurse	Nurse-physician

2. **To establish a partnership the partners must agree to the following statements:**
   - We're both clear about our joint purpose, and we're both responsible.*
   - I can be trusted; I promise to be honest.
   - We're each responsible for our own emotional well-being (if I feel bad about something, it's my responsibility to do something about it)*
   - We should make decisions together as much as possible.
   - We both have the right to say no, so long as no harm is done.*
   - We'll both agree to rules for resolving conflict between us.
   - We both can expect to grow and learn from our experience.
   - I choose to be here, so nobody's to blame.*
   - We're both responsible for the outcomes (consequences) of our actions.
   - If one of us sees the other engage in unsafe or unethical conduct, we have the responsibility to address it appropriately.

---

*In the context of the nurse-patient relationship, these statements aren't completely true: Nurses often must be held more responsible than patients. Nurses don't have the right to say no if it jeopardizes patients' health (they must find a replacement). Patients often have few choices about where they are.

3. **An empowered partnership requires choosing to:**
   - Rise to the challenge of taking charge over the comfort of remaining dependent.
   - Give up some of the power, take calculated, thoughtful risks, and be willing to do the work needed to be independent.

4. **An empowered partnership also requires*:**
   - Nonjudgmental acceptance.
   - Space for self-expression.
   - Structure for conflict resolution.
   - Respect for each other's boundaries.
   - Support and encouragement for the growth in the areas where one is limited.
   - Transformation coaching (coaching that truly affects the learner's attitudes and skills).
   - Growth of partners.

5. **Many people are uncomfortable in an empowered partnership** for the following reasons:
   - They are used to being taken care of and aren't accustomed to taking responsibility.
   - They are unwilling to accept the responsibility that comes with power.
   - They are unwilling to give up some of the power they're accustomed to having.
   - They haven't made the required shift in thinking (they don't truly believe in the benefits of partnership).

6. **Change takes time.** Gently coach those who aren't accustomed to the roles and responsibilities of being in a partnership.

 OTHER PERSPECTIVES

Patients As Partners

"Patients have to be partners, equally responsible for treatment."

—Tommy LaSorta, former Los Angeles Dodgers manager

Teacher Student Partnerships

"[Many students believe] 'teacher knows what's best for me.' We think that the task of these leaders is to create an environment where we can live a life of safety and predictability. Dependency also holds those above us responsible for how we feel about ourselves (we want that positive feedback)."[†]

—Peter Block, Author and Consultant

---

*Block, P. (1996). *Stewardship: Choosing service over self-interest.* San Francisco, CA: Berrett-Koehler, p. 29.

†Ibid. p. 37.

Related Skills: Giving and Taking Feedback (below), Managing Conflicts Constructively (page 205).

Critical Thinking Exercises

Instructions: In a group, in a personal journal, or both:

1. Discuss how establishing partnerships with peers is different from establishing partnerships with patients.
2. Address how establishing an empowered partnership is affected by:
   - The length of contact you have with a patient.
   - The patient's health state.
   - Growth and development (e.g., How do you partner with a child or an elderly person?).
3. Explain what is meant by, Partnership is an attitude as much as a model for relationships.
4. Ask a peer to partner with you in completing a course or accomplishing a goal. Agree from the beginning to follow the strategies listed in this section.
5. Determine whether you can achieve the Learning Outcomes at the beginning of this skill.

References

Block, P. (1996). *Stewardship: Choosing service over self-interest.* San Francisco, CA: Berrett-Koehler.

Heinemann, D., Lengacher, C., Vancott, M., Mabe, P., Swymer, S. (1996). Partners in patient care: Measuring the effect on patient satisfaction and other quality indicators. *Nursing Economics, 14*, 278–285.

Paul, S. (1998). The advanced practice/staff nurse partnership: Building a winning team. *Critical Care Nurse, 18*(2), 92–97.

5. GIVING AND TAKING FEEDBACK

Definition

Being able to provide and accept constructive criticism.

Learning Outcomes

After you study this information and complete the accompanying exercises you should be able to:

- Discuss the effect of emotional responses to criticism.
- Determine how you can improve your response to criticism.
- Identify strategies for giving constructive criticism.

Thinking Critically about Feedback

How we think and behave is an extremely complex issue that's closely linked to self-esteem. Being told we could be a better thinker, improve in some way, or approach things differently often brings up intensely uncomfortable feelings of being wrong or not good enough. These gut reactions cloud key issues and paralyze our ability to be objective. Knowing how to provide constructive criticism in a supportive way can make the difference between alienating others and motivating them to improve. Knowing how to accept criticism—to be objective and work through the negative aspects of criticism—reduces our stress and helps us grow.

Strategies for Giving and Taking Feedback*

1. **Giving feedback**
   - Be sensitive to personality differences (personalities of both the giver and the receiver greatly affect feedback).
   - Keep in mind that without mutual trust, feedback is unlikely to be viewed constructively.
   - Give feedback frequently and in a timely way (this way it's viewed as being more sincere).
   - Separate negative and positive feedback as much as possible. When you sandwich positive and negative in one statement, it dilutes the effects of both.
   - Start with what's being done right (for example, Here are the things I see that you're doing right); then focus on what *could be improved* (rather than on what's *wrong*).
   - Remain fully engaged in the communication; listen actively to avoid misunderstandings and making false assumptions.

---

*Adapted from Musinski, B. Unpublished Workshop handouts.

- Give positive feedback often to reward growth (for example, "catch" people being effective and surprise them with positive feedback).
- Be aware that too much negative feedback can hinder progress by making the person afraid of failure.
- Learn how to be assertive without being aggressive (see Box 6–2, below).

BOX 6–2 **Being Assertive Without Being Aggressive***

Assertive behavior means:

- Expressing your feelings, ideas, and needs calmly and openly.
- Standing up for your own rights while showing respect for the rights of others.
- Confronting fairly, being sensitive to when others feel threatened.
- Valuing yourself; acting with confidence.
- Owning responsibility and speaking with authority.
- Building equal relationships and finding common goals.

Using assertive behavior:

1. Accept the anger or discomfort you may have as your own; do not blame others. You own the problem!
   - Identify the key components of the situation and how you feel about them.
   - How do you think others who are involved feel about the issue?
   - Decide which of your needs were not met.
2. Be cognizant of your own behavior; keep a lid on your emotions (no easy task!).
3. Meet privately with the person(s); listen before you speak.
4. Use assertive listening (this is an intellectual function that requires patience, hard work, and practice).
   - Actively commit to the other person; concentrate your attention so you accurately hear feelings, opinions, and wishes.
   - Try to understand completely before responding.
   - Paraphrase what the other person(s) have said to be sure you understand.
5. State your own feelings, thoughts, and needs clearly, in a nonthreatening way.
   - Use eye contact, a direct body posture, and a controlled voice volume and tone.
   - Using "I" messages, be clear about behavior that disturbs you and how you feel (for example, I was very embarrassed and hurt when I saw you walk away from our conversation. Rather than, You made me feel like such a jerk when. . . .).

*Adapted from Musinski, B. (1998). Unpublished Workshop handouts.

2. Accepting feedback

- Pay attention to how your emotions are affecting your ability to use the feedback in a positive way. For example, say to yourself, I'm getting upset. I'd better take a deep breath, calm down, and listen. If I work to remain objective and not take things personally, I might learn something when I think about this later when I'm less stressed.* Befriend criticism, evaluating it objectively. Someone wanted you to succeed or would not have bothered to share their thoughts.
- Ask yourself, Have I heard this same criticism from other people? If so, it's most likely true.
- Keep in mind that not all criticism is given constructively, but try to focus on what you can learn.
- If you agree with the criticism, acknowledge that the critic is right and begin to think about what you can do about it.
- Don't make excuses for yourself, don't be defensive, and sincerely try to see the benefits of the criticism.
- Practice personal feedback by monitoring your own behavior and paying attention to how others respond to you.
- Don't let false pride, rationalization, or other negative factors get in the way of your growth.
- Remember that no one's perfect, but we can all improve. Be prepared to expend some physical and emotional energy to change.

 OTHER PERSPECTIVES

Deal With It

"Feedback is important. It helps us stay focused and on course. We all need to know how to give it, take it, deal with it, and accept it."   —*Barbara A. Musinski, RNC, BS*

Related Skills: Managing Conflict Constructively (page 205).

Critical Thinking Exercises

Instructions: In a group, in a personal journal, or both:

---

*Adapted from Weisinger, H. (1998). *Emotional intelligence at work.* San Francisco, CA: Jossey-Bass.

1. Think about a time you tried to give feedback to someone to help him or her improve. Describe what happened and how you felt at the time. What, if anything, would you do differently if you had to do it again?
2. Think about a time someone gave you feedback. Explain what happened and how you felt at the time. Then follow up with your thoughts on the matter today. For example, what made things easier or harder? What did you learn in the long run?
3. Think about the following statement and decide what you would do if you had to give feedback to someone you don't get along with. *Without mutual trust, feedback is unlikely to be viewed constructively.*
4. Determine whether you can achieve the Learning Outcomes at the beginning of this skill.

References

Alberti, R., Emmons, M. (1988). *Your perfect right, a guide to assertive living.* San Luis Obispo, CA: Impact Publishers.

Cadwell, C. (1995). *Powerful performance appraisals.* Franklin Lakes, NJ: Career Press.

Paulson, T. (1991). *They shoot managers, don't they?* Berkeley, CA: Ten Speed Press.

Rager, P. (1998). Emotional intelligence and the management edge. *Nursing Spectrum (FL ED), 8*(3), 3.

Weisinger, H. (1998). *Emotional intelligence at work.* San Francisco, CA: Jossey-Bass.

Weisinger, H., Lobsenz, N. (1983). *Nobody's perfect.* New York: Warner Books.

6. MANAGING CONFLICT CONSTRUCTIVELY

Definition

Being able to make conflict work in positive ways (learning, growth, improvement).

Background Information. Conflict can be severe, taking the form of sharp disagreement and fighting, or it can be mild, taking the form of subtle, even subconscious opposition to an idea or action. For many, the word "conflict" has negative connotations, bringing feelings of discomfort and dread. Most of us deeply want to live in a world where everyone gets along and everything goes smoothly. However, in this age of dealing with complex issues, conflict is a *normal* part of every relationship and project—without it you're unlikely to grow and improve.

Learning Outcomes

After you study this information and complete the accompanying exercises you should be able to:

- Identify your usual approach to dealing with conflict.
- Determine strategies to improve your ability to make conflict work in positive ways.

Thinking Critically about Conflict

Critical thinking requires being able to understand and exchange different viewpoints, wants, and needs and to come to a sincere agreement about what's most important. Knowing how to make conflict work in positive ways helps you seize opportunities for growth and to achieve realistic outcomes that are more likely to work. When you're comfortable and skilled in recognizing and managing conflict, you have more brain power to focus on making real progress—you reduce the amount of time and energy spent dealing with the negative outcomes of conflict (see Table 6–2).

TABLE 6–2	**Outcomes of Conflict**
NEGATIVE OUTCOMES OF CONFLICT	POSITIVE OUTCOMES OF MANAGING CONFLICT CONSTRUCTIVELY
Increased stress	Reduced stress
Decreased productivity	Increased harmony and productivity
Poor relationships/feelings of isolation	Better relationships/more interaction
	Better understanding of others involved
Wasted time and energy	Improved ability to clarify main issues/find creative solutions
Frustration, anger, hopelessness	Improved self-steem
Lack of growth	Opportunity to improve bothersome things
Poor self-esteem	

Strategies for Managing Conflict Constructively

There are five key steps to mastering the skill of managing conflict constructively:

1. **Gain insight into your natural style of dealing with conflict (Box 6–3).** Make a commitment to consciously work to draw

---

BOX 6–3   **Managing Conflict: What's Your Style?**

AVOIDERS pull away. They ignore issues or withdraw from people they feel are causing conflict. Avoiders often get along well with others because they focus on promoting peace and harmony. However, they tend to allow problems to persist and place little importance on their own needs. As a result, they miss opportunities to make improvements and tend to "explode" when things finally get to be too much, even though the trigger issue may be minor.

ACCOMMODATORS/SMOOTHERS give up their own needs and try to make others feel better. This group often struggles with inner conflicts because they secretly wish to speak their minds. They too can explode, damaging relationships because of failure to honestly confront issues that are important to them.

FORCERS try to get THEIR way even if it means others have to give up what they want or need. They're minimally interested in or aware of what others need and don't really care if they are liked.

COMPROMISERS give up part of their wants and needs and persuade others to give up part of their wants and needs. They think they get win-win solutions but may be settling for minimally acceptable solutions that continue the conflict (because they assume everyone has to lose something in negotiations rather than persisting to find answers that fully satisfy everyone involved).

COLLABORATIVE PROBLEM SOLVERS make it a rule to fairly face issues together. This group has equal concern for both the issues and the relationship. They see conflict as a means of improving relationships by gaining understanding and reducing tension. They look for solutions that allow everyone to win by identifying areas of agreement and differences, evaluating alternatives, and choosing solutions that have the full support of the key parties involved.

Summary

Collaborating = win-win.

Compromising = win a little, lose a little (sometimes unavoidable).

Avoiding = lose-lose (sometimes may be used *purposely* to buy time, which is an appropriate use of this strategy).

Accommodating = one side consistently loses so the other has its way.

Forcing = one side consistently wins, while the other loses.

upon strengths and work on weaknesses in an objective, purposeful manner.

2. **Learn how to recognize patterns and appearances of conflict** *early.* Become cognizant of verbal and nonverbal behaviors that signal conflict may be developing (e.g., withdrawal, verbalization of problems with current state of affairs).

3. **Practice using conflict management strategies (Box 6–4).**

4. **Develop skills you need to function more comfortably when faced with conflict** (e.g., being assertive without being aggressive, see Box 6–2).

5. **Use a comprehensive approach to assessing and managing conflict:**
   - Hold opinions until you're sure of all the facts.
   - Choose an appropriate time and place to open discussion (ensure privacy and find a convenient time for those involved).
   - Be willing to persevere until you clearly understand the issues, values, and goals of the key players involved.
   - Foster an atmosphere of trust and sincere desire to face issues fairly together; encourage free exchange of ideas, feelings, and attitudes.
   - Stay focused on common values and goals; look for win-win solutions (some compromising may be needed).
   - Look for several solutions to the problems, evaluating each solution with the key players involved.
   - Make a conscious effort to stay calm, help others stay calm, and keep the focus on the positive outcomes of resolving the conflict.
   - Take a break or get help from outside sources as needed. Allow for time out but keep interacting until all parties agree to the solution.
   - Set up a time to revisit issues to see if the solutions are actually being carried out and helping reduce the problem.

6. Apply principles of negotiation as needed (see Box 6–5).

 OTHER PERSPECTIVES

Mustering up Courage

"Confrontation takes considerable courage, and many people would rather take the course of least resistance, belittling and criticizing, betraying confidences, or participating in gossip about others behind their backs. But in the long run, people will trust and respect you if you are honest and open and kind with them. You care enough to confront."*

—Stephen Covey, Author and Leadership Coach

---

*Covey, S. (1989). *The seven habits of highly effective people.* New York: Simon & Schuster, p. 157.

BOX 6-4   **Mad about You: Managing Conflict Constructively**

- **Listen with the intent to understand** the other parties' points of view before presenting your own.
- **Keep a lid on your emotions.** It's hard to think clearly when your adrenaline is flowing.
- **Using "I" messages** and a nonthreatening tone of voice clearly explain how the problem is affecting you and what you'd like to happen.
  - I feel (name the feeling).
  - When I see/hear (state the problem).
  - I would like (state the change you want to happen).
- **Ask yourself, What can I find in this situation that I'm doing to contribute to the problem?** You have more control over things that *you're* doing to contribute to the problem than over things that *others* are doing to contribute to the problem.
- **Get rid of old baggage** (feelings and preconceptions you have because of things that have happened in the past). For example, thinking, I'm just not the type of person who can handle conflict, so she knows she can get her way.
- **Look for deep issues.** For example, say, Tell me what's really bothering you (keep repeating this if the answer is, I don't know).
- **Be willing to hear things you don't like to hear**. You need honest feedback to work through the issues.
- **Ask for help from those involved.** For example, Can we agree to not be so hard on one another?
- **Change your approach** to managing conflict depending on the situation rather than using the style you're most comfortable with. For example, one survey revealed that on the whole, nurses use *avoidance* as a primary style for resolving conflicts. The second and third most frequently used styles are *compromise* and *accommodation.** All three styles may involve more losing than necessary.
  - **Use collaborative problem solving** as the overall, optimum way to manage conflict. Because this approach takes more time than you may have at the moment, initially you may need to use one of the following approaches. You also may need to use all the methods below as stepping stones to collaborative problem solving.
  - **Use avoidance** only when trying to delay confrontation until a more appropriate time, when time out is required, or when issues are of minor importance in relation to overall goal.
  - **Use accommodation/smoothing** when the goal is to preserve relationships or encourage the others to express themselves.
  - **Use compromise** when time is too limited for a full collaborative approach and there are two equally empowered sides who must maintain a positive relationship yet reach agreement. Find a common ground to achieve temporary settlement that at least satisfies each side's main objectives.
  - **Use forcing** only when there isn't time for discussion (e.g., an emergency), when you must implement unpopular changes, or when all other strategies have failed and the change is required.

*Restifo, V. (1996). Surviving and thriving with conflict on the job. *Nursing Spectrum (PA ED)*, 5(2), 12.

BOX 6–5	**How to Negotiate***

Negotiation requires:

- Being clear about what results you want to achieve.
- Building and maintaining a communication climate that supports problem solving under stress.
- Letting other parties know your interests and actively working to discover theirs.
- A willingness to explore the needs of all parties and a determination to use problem-solving skills to find mutually agreeable solutions.
- Determining *common interests* as well as conflicting needs and desires.
- Being willing to think about various proposals and making a decision about whether to reject, reframe, or accept them.
- Knowing your BATNA (Best Alternative To a Negotiated Agreement). A BATNA is like a worst-case scenario. It's the lowest level of what you're willing to accept. Reject any offer that falls below this level. Consider and discuss any offer that's less than you'd like but better than your BATNA.

*Data from Glaser, R. (1994). *Building negotiating power.* King of Prussia, PA: Organization Design and Development, pp. 3–7.

CRITICAL MOMENTS

Adrenaline Rush Clouds Thinking

Ever notice how hard it is to stay calm and objective when faced with conflict? The fight or flight response easily initiated by threats to self causes our adrenal glands to inject adrenaline into the blood stream, bringing a rush of emotion and excitement that makes it harder to think clearly. When faced with conflict, give yourself and others time to calm down and think things through.

Related Skills: Communicating Bad News (page 192), Giving and Taking Feedback (page 201).

Critical Thinking Exercises

1. **Gain insight into how you tend to respond to conflict and how you feel about others' styles for resolving conflict.** In a group, in a personal journal, or both:
   a. List three or four conflicts that you can remember in some detail.
   b. Review the styles in Box 6–3 and honestly consider what styles you used while in conflict. Once you've considered your own

style, think about what styles the other person(s) used and how they affected you.

c. Now that time has passed, imagine how you could have handled the situation better or what style(s) may have achieved a better outcome.

2. Choose one or two of the preceding situations and share them with a partner or in a group, asking for a different viewpoint on what was going on in the conflict and what styles and strategies might have been helpful.

3. **Practice using "I" messages.** Change the following statements to ones that send "I" messages.

   a. You never listen to me.
   b. I wish you wouldn't be so sloppy all the time.
   c. You make me feel like I'm the one who causes all the problems.
   d. You make me feel insignificant when you ignore me like that.
   e. Why are you always attacking me?

4. **Imagine this:** Someone tells you one of your patients has numerous complaints. You go directly to the room, knock, introduce yourself, and inquire about the problem. The patient's wife immediately becomes hostile and tells you to "just get out." What do you do? Explain your rationale.

5. **Use role playing to practice assertive communication and conflict resolution.** Get a partner. Have one of you be the manager in the following situation and the other be the staff nurse. Here's the situation:

   A staff nurse is angry because he didn't get a specific day off, even though he had put in a written request well ahead of time. He needs the weekend off for his daughter's birthday. The manager spent hours trying to find proper coverage but couldn't honor his request because two other nurses also needed to be off and had been turned down for their requests the previous month.

6. Evaluate whether you can achieve the Learning Outcomes at the beginning of this section.

References

Alberti, R., Emmons, M. (1988). *Your perfect right, a guide to assertive living.* San Luis Obispo, CA: Impact Publishers.

Blickensderfer, L. (1993). Assertive communication. *Nursing Spectrum (FL ED), 3*(2), 13–15.

Erwin, K. (1992). Managing conflict. *Nursing Management, 23*(3), 67.

Glaser, R. (1994). *Building negotiating power.* King of Prussia, PA: Organization Design and Development, pp. 3–7.

Restifo, V. (1996). Surviving and thriving with conflict on the job. *Nursing Spectrum (PA ED), 5*(2), 12–13.

Shaskin, M. (1989). *Managing conflict constructively.* King of Prussia, PA: Organization Design and Development.

Weisinger, H. (1998). *Emotional intelligence at work.* San Francisco, CA: Jossey-Bass.

Wolf, Z., Brennan, R., Ferchau, L., Magee, M., et al. (1997). Creating and implementing guidelines on caring for difficult patients: A research utilization project. *MEDSURG NURSING, 6*(3), 137–147.

7. PREVENTING AND DEALING WITH MISTAKES CONSTRUCTIVELY

Definition

Knowing how to prevent, detect, correct, and learn from errors.

Background Information. Mistakes can be our worst nightmare, or they can be stepping stones to learning and improvement. And sometimes, they can be both. Dealing with mistakes is a complex issue that includes considering legal consequences. This section is intended to give beginning insight into dealing with mistakes. It addresses how to know what constitutes a serious error, why errors happen, and how to prevent, detect, correct, and learn from errors.

Learning Outcomes

After you study this information and complete the accompanying exercises you should be able to:

- Explain how to determine the seriousness of a mistake.
- Identify circumstances that lead you to make mistakes.
- Develop a personal plan for preventing, detecting, correcting, and learning from mistakes.

Thinking Critically about Mistakes

Too many people have a one-size-fits-all mindset when it comes to dealing with mistakes. Deep down they believe that all errors are bad, that all errors happen because of lack of knowledge or laziness, and that the best way to deal with those who make errors is to punish them. However, this approach shames those involved, doesn't examine the real causes of errors, and does little to reduce the incidence of mistakes. The reality is that many mistakes happen for multiple reasons and in spite of good intentions. Changing the mindset from "mistakes shouldn't happen" to "when dealing with humans, *mistakes will* happen for various reasons" can help us identify specific strategies tailored to reduce the likelihood of negative outcomes. Box 6–6 shows four common reasons medication errors happen.

Strategies for Preventing and Dealing with Mistakes Constructively

1. **Determine how serious the error is.** Serious errors need to be examined more closely, prevented more meticulously, and detected and corrected more quickly than less serious errors.

   ■ **Rule: To determine the seriousness of a mistake:** Decide *what harm could result* if the error happens (primarily consider harm in terms of human morbidity, mortality, and suffering; secondarily consider harm in terms of inconvenience, cost, and lost time). If you're unable to decide what harm could result, ask for help.

BOX 6–6	**Four Common Reasons Why Medication Errors Happen***

1. **Inadequate knowledge and skill:** These reflect lack of patient knowledge, patient's diagnosis, and the names, purposes, and correct administration of medications.
2. **Failure to comply with policies and procedures:** Lack of attention to safeguards in medication administration procedures intended to prevent errors.
3. **Communication failure:** These include transcription errors, use of abbreviations, illegible handwriting, incorrect interpretation of physician's orders, use of verbal orders, failure to record medications given or omitted, and unclear medication administration records.
4. **Individual and system problems:** These include things like the number of years of experience of the nurse, number of consecutive hours worked, rotating shifts, workload, distractions and interruptions, floating nurses to unfamiliar units, hospital and pharmacy design features, and drug manufacturing problems (e.g., look-alike and sound-alike drug names, look-alike packaging, confusing and unclear labeling, failure to specify drug concentrations on dose-calculation charts).

*Data from Wakefield, B., Wakefield, D., Uden-Holdman, T., Blegen, M. (1998). Nurses' perception of why medication administration errors occur. *MEDSURG Nursing, 7*(1), 39–44.

Example of a serious error: You forget to check someone's identification bracelet before sending him to the operating room. **Example of a less serious error:** While inserting a Foley catheter, you contaminate the package and have to get a new one.

2. **Become familiar with the following common types of errors and how to prevent them:**
   - **Mental slip:** These mistakes happen when there's a lapse in your attention to what you're doing or when there's a lapse in short-term memory. *Example:* You're on the way to check an IV, but you're interrupted to help lift someone up in bed. After you finish helping, you forget that you were on the way to check the IV and go on to another task. *Prevention:* Keeping a personal worksheet that prompts you to do important tasks (e.g., check IV every hour) can help you catch mental slips early. Getting charting done as soon as possible also helps you notice when you've forgotten to do something. Checklists, protocols, and computerized decision aides all help reduce mental slips because they relieve you from relying on short-term memory, a part of memory that becomes most imperfect under stress or fatigue.
   - **Interaction error:** These mistakes happen when people misunderstand each other. *Example:* You're working in the emergency department and have been talking to Dr. French about one of the patients, Mrs. Moran. A few minutes later, Dr. French comes to you and says, "Would you send her to x-ray?" nodding in the direction of another patient. You don't see him nod in the other direction and assume Dr. French is referring to Mrs. Moran. *Prevention:* Repeating what you think you heard also helps clarify verbal interactions (e.g., You want me to send Mrs. Moran to x-ray?). Always checking written orders clarifies verbal orders.
   - **Knowledge error:** These mistakes are due to insufficient knowledge. *Example:* You cause unnecessary side effects by giving IV drug too quickly because you didn't know it should be given slowly. *Prevention:* Be sure you know the answers to who, what, why, when, and how *in the context of each individual patient situation* before you give any drug or perform any intervention.
   - **Learning error:** Although these mistakes often include knowledge errors, learning errors are often related to several different factors associated with being in a learning situation (e.g.,

doing something for the first time, having less than astute observation skills, being stressed). *Example:* You're changing sterile dressings for the first time. You contaminate your glove by slightly touching an unsterile field. You don't notice it because you're focusing on assessing the wound. *Prevention:* A sure-fire way to avoid learning errors is not to try anything new, which makes no sense. Many students hide from new experiences because they're afraid of making mistakes, which doesn't work either because it just postpones the inevitable. The best way to avoid learning errors is to be prepared and to practice, practice, practice in as safe an environment as possible (e.g., skills lab). In risky situations it's best to have a more experienced nurse observe learner performance, give advice, or actually handle the task at hand.

- **Overreliance on technology:** These mistakes happen when you rely too much on technology, without using your human capabilities. *Example:* Someone complains that a heating pad is too hot, but when you check it, you find that it's on the low setting. Rather than carefully feeling the pad yourself, you explain that it's probably okay because it's set on low. *Prevention:* Read all instruction manuals carefully. Don't trust machines more than your own knowledge and perceptions.

- **System error:** These mistakes are usually considered from a big-picture perspective. In other words, these mistakes are related to something wrong with the way things are accomplished within the facility as a whole. *Examples:* Drugs that aren't given because the pharmacist is overloaded and unable to dispense the drug in a timely manner; errors that happen because a policy or procedure is unclear; errors that happen because a facility uses a lot of per diem personnel who are more at risk for making mistakes. *Prevention:* Report possible system problems to the risk management or quality assurance department. Create a multidisciplinary panel to examine possible and actual system problems.

3. **Follow policies and procedures and be sure you understand the rationale behind them.** These are designed by experts to prevent, detect, and correct errors early.

4. **When using checklists, focus on each item carefully.** Checklists are supposed to jog your brain, not replace it.

5. **Involve patients and families in their own health care as much as possible.** Educate them and encourage them to become active

partners with their caregivers in preventing errors by verifying that they're getting the right treatments and medications.

6. **Never perform an intervention without being sure you clearly understand why it's indicated in each particular situation.**

7. **Be careful about multitasking.** Trying to do too many things at once predisposes you to omitting something important.

8. **Involve experts.** For example, if confused about a medication regimen, ask a pharmacist; include experts from several disciplines or areas on error prevention initiatives.

9. **Look after yourself.** When you know how to deal with stress and are rested and alert, you're less likely to make mistakes.

10. **When a mistake happens:**
    - Rank the seriousness of the error as soon as it's recognized (see rule on page 213).
    - Immediately address the error to prevent or reduce harm.
    - Chart actions taken to address the error (e.g., increased monitoring, transfer to another unit, etc.)
    - Follow policy and procedures for dealing with mistakes.
    - Curb the tendency to focus too much on guilt and not enough on what can be learned from your own perspective and from the perspective of other students and nurses.
    - Explore the specifics of the incident objectively and scrutinize the procedures leading to the errors. Consider the value of sharing the mistake with others to alert them of the possibility of its happening again. If procedures were followed and a mistake still happened, maybe the procedures should be revised to make them more error proof.

◼ **Want to Know More?** Visit the web page of the National Patient Safety Foundation (http://www.ama-assn.org/med-sci/npsf/main.htm) or email questions to npsf@ama-assn.org. They gather and disseminate information about the causes and responses to error, with the goal of increasing patient safety by developing tools to prevent mistakes.

CRITICAL MOMENT

Do Not Disturb

Pilots have a "sterile" cockpit. During a specific period of time before landing and after take-off, no one is to enter the cockpit, and cockpit conversation is limited to flight procedures only. To ensure that this is so, pilots' conversations are recorded. Nurses can learn from pilots. During crucial moments, like preparing medications, ask not to be disturbed, and don't disturb others.

OTHER PERSPECTIVES

Research Raises Questions About Med Errors

"[Research findings] support the notion that medication administration is more than a simple psychomotor task. It's a complex process involving multiple interactions among professionals, patients, and the health care environment. . . . It's critical that this complex process be analyzed and improved. [The findings of our] study raise a number of important nursing research and management questions. How inter- and intra-professional relationships and conflict contribute to causing medication administration errors is perhaps the biggest unanswered question. The effects of computerized systems on prescribing practices, medication administration documentation, and error reporting and analysis is another important area of investigation. . . . Clearly, much more can and should be done to 'change the system' and change individual behaviors to prevent future medication errors."*

Related Skills: Communicating Bad News (page 192).

Critical Thinking Exercises

Instructions: In a group, in a personal journal, or both:

1. Address the implications of the following statements.
   - To be ignorant doesn't merely mean not to know; it means not to know what you don't know; being educated means knowing precisely what you don't know.
   - As a nurse it's your responsibility to be alert not only to situations that might cause *you* to make a mistake but also to situations that may cause *others* to make a mistake.
2. Read the Other Perspectives on page 218. Then explore:
   - How you feel when you make a mistake.
   - What you can do to help someone else who has made a mistake.
   - Ways to correct systems and increase checks to prevent medication errors.

---

*From Wakefield, B., Wakefield, D., Uden-Holdman, T., Blegen, M. (1998). Nurses' perception of why medication administration errors occur. *MEDSURG Nursing, 7*(1), 39–44.

OTHER PERSPECTIVES

No One's Perfect

"A system designed for safety is one based on the assumption that errors will be made. [Those] working in hospitals must recognize that mistakes will be made and plan for their quick remediation. Systems should be designed, constructed, maintained, and used in ways that preclude any possibility for error. Healthcare is similar to the aviation industry in that human error accounts for a significant proportion of preventable negative outcomes, but the error is encased in situations involving complex equipment and multiple interactions. Despite the airline industry's remarkable safety record over the past 75 years, pilot errors are common. For example, on international flights the pilot or crew makes an error every 4 minutes on the average. However, these errors don't result in serious problems or crashes because flight protocols and the electronic systems are designed so that errors are quickly recognized and corrected.*

3. Pick any three issues of the *American Journal of Nursing* and summarize the "Med Error" section.
4. Determine whether you can achieve the Learning Outcomes at the beginning of this skill.

References

Boivin, J. (1997). There's no room for error. *Nursing Spectrum (FL ED), 7*(7), 3, 17.

Eskreis, T. (1998). Seven common legal pitfalls in nursing. *American Journal of Nursing, 98*(4), 34–41.

Wakefield, B., Wakefield, D., Uden-Holdman, T., Blegen, M. (1998). Nurses' perception of why medication administration errors occur. *MEDSURG Nursing, 7*(1), 39–44.

Wolf, Z. (1994). *Medication errors: The nursing experience.* Albany, NY: Delmar.

---

*From Dracup, K., Bryan-Brown, C. (1996). Making mistakes (editorial). *American Journal of Critical Care, 5*(1), 2.

8. TRANSFORMING A GROUP INTO A TEAM

Definition

Knowing how to work together harmoniously to combine efforts to achieve shared outcomes within a specific time frame.

Learning Outcomes

After you study this information and complete the accompanying exercises you should be able to:

- Explain the common stages of team building.
- Describe strategies that transform groups into teams.
- Participate more effectively as part of a team.

Thinking Critically about Teamwork

Whether you're working in the clinical area, on a committee, or on a group project, teamwork doesn't just happen. It must be nurtured as it evolves, using approaches that help transform a diverse group into a harmonious team.

True teamwork occurs when all team members are:
- Committed to common goals and a high level of output.
- Energized by their ability to work together.
- Concerned about how team members feel during the work process.

For example, consider the difference between what's going on in groups A and B below.

Group A consists of several nurses who have been working together for the past 6 months. They don't feel like they're working together as a team and wonder what they can do to correct the situation. Their manager is a busy person who happens to have a demanding boss. When the pressure is on, she barks orders and personally takes over some tasks. The staff responds by doing what they are told or lying low until things calm down. Group participation in problem solving and decision making is almost nonexistent. Most of the nurses want to perform their responsibilities in a satisfactory way. But they have never given much thought to the need for group goals or concerted group action. Under these circumstances it seems nothing will change, morale is low, and everyone dreads coming to work.

Group B consists of several nurses who also have been working together for 6 months in a situation similar to that of group A. By contrast these nurses are energized and proud of their successes. Like group A, their manager also is a busy person with a demanding boss. However, when the pressure is on, she stops the action, convenes a problem-solving discussion, focusing on common goals and getting input from team members. The result is that better solutions are found because the pressure is channeled into a spirit of let's fix this together. These nurses enjoy a sense of growing and improving together—work is more than just a job.*

Strategies for Transforming a Group into a Team

1. All those involved should remember the importance of using behaviors that enhance interpersonal relationships (see Table 6–3).
2. **Team *leaders* should:**
   - Create a shared vision of the team's mission or purpose: everyone must be committed to reaching clearly defined outcomes.
   - Stress that everyone is responsible for improving performance by scrutinizing practices and pointing out improvements that could be made.
   - Turn diversity to the team's advantage (e.g., assign tasks based on individual strengths and preferences as much as possible).
   - Ask for consensus in decisions (everyone agrees to agree), rather than settling for a majority vote.
   - Be careful not to criticize ideas.
   - Keep team members well informed so that everyone has a good understanding of the big picture.
   - Recognize team members for their contribution.
   - Be sure team members are familiar with the common stages of team building (see Box 6–7, page 222). Although not every group goes through every stage, and length of time for each stage varies, it helps to know that there are common struggles in every team.
3. **Team *members* should:**
   - Agree about roles, responsibilities, and proper lines of communication.
   - Get involved and contribute to the good of the group.

---

*Adapted from *Building a Winning Team* © 1994 by Dr. Rollin Glaser and Christine Glaser with permission of Organization Design and Development Inc., King of Prussia, Pennsylvania, p. 2.

TABLE 6–3	Behaviors Enhancing and Impeding Interpersonal Relationships*

BEHAVIORS THAT ENHANCE INTERPERSONAL RELATIONSHIPS	BEHAVIORS THAT INHIBIT INTERPERSONAL RELATIONSHIPS
• Conveying an attitude of openness, acceptance, and lack of prejudice.	• Conveying an attitude of doubt, mistrust, or negative judgment.
• Being honest.	• Giving false information.
• Taking initiative and responsibility.	• Conveying an "it's not my job" attitude.
• Being reliable.	• Not meeting commitments, only partially meeting commitments, or not being punctual.
• Demonstrating humility.	• Demonstrating self-importance.
• Showing respect for what others are, have been, or may become.	• "Talking down," or assuming familiarity.
• Accepting accountability.	• Making excuses or placing blame where it doesn't belong.
• Being confident and prepared.	• Being unsure and trying to "wing it."
• Showing genuine interest.	• Acting like you're only doing something because it's a job.
• Conveying appreciation for others' time.	• Assuming others have more time than we do.
• Accepting expression of positive *and* negative feelings.	• Demonstrating annoyance when negative feelings are expressed.
• Taking enough time.	• Rushing.
• Being frank and forthright.	• Sending mixed messages, saying things just because we think it's what the other person wants to hear, or talking behind others' backs.
• Admitting when we've been wrong.	• Denying or ignoring when we've made an error.
• Apologizing if we've caused distress or inconvenience.	• Acting like nothing happened or making excuses.

*Adapted with permission from Alfaro-LeFevre, R. (1998). *Applying nursing process: A step by step guide* (4th ed.). Philadelphia: J.B. Lippincott.

BOX 6–7	**Common Stages of Team Building**

Forming

Group members start to get to know one another, testing each other's values, beliefs, and attitudes. Basic goals and tasks are defined, roles assigned, and ideas shared.

Storming

Conflict within begins, often because of misunderstandings or disagreement about *what* realistically can get done and *how* exactly things will get done. More testing goes on in this phase, with some people asking themselves questions like, How much am I willing to do? This is a time to maintain high standards, provide emotional support, and aim to get consensus (agreement from everyone). Beware of false consensus during this phase—some people will say they agree when they really *don't* (just to avoid further conflict). Because this is a stressful stage, you may need to take more breaks.

Norming

The group becomes more cohesive and really wants to work together in positive way. Group members agree on rules—for example, when meetings will be held, who should attend, what proper lines of communication are, and how problems and disagreements will be handled. At this point the leader needs to be sensitive to group values, asking for votes to determine common needs and desires.

Performing

Team members begin to bond to one another and function well together with a good understanding of role, responsibilities, and relationships.

- Stay focused on the big picture of what the team is trying to accomplish.
- Remember to listen actively.
- Make a conscious effort to overcome the human tendency to focus narrowly on self—too often team members who feel very responsible have difficulty seeing other members' struggles because they themselves are working so hard.
- Stress the need for all to model behaviors that promote trust and create a caring and energized environment.

- Follow the Golden Rule—point out when it's not being followed (without blaming).
- Show enthusiasm—it's contagious and energizes others.
- Be clear on what's expected of you; work hard to be good at what you do; and deliver what you promise.
- Address and resolve conflicts early—push for high-quality communication.
- Be aware of group process and where the team is in relation to the stages of team building (see Box 6–7).
- Recognize individual and team efforts; be a good sport.
- Help new teammates make entry.
- Support creativity and new ways of doing things.
- Broaden your skills; offer to try new tasks or to cross train.
- Promote group learning by collecting, sharing, and analyzing information.
- Spend fun time together (here's where relationships grow).

 OTHER PERSPECTIVES

Do You See Yourself as Part of Something Bigger?

"[There's a story] about a little wave, bobbing along in the ocean, having a grand old time. He's enjoying the wind and the fresh air—until he notices the other waves in front of him crashing against the shore.

"'My God, this is terrible,' the wave says. 'Look what's going to happen to me!'

"Then along comes another wave. It sees the first wave looking grim, and it says to him, 'Why do you look so sad?'

"The first wave says, 'You don't understand! We're all going to crash! All of us waves are going to be nothing! Isn't it terrible?'

"The second wave says, 'No, *you* don't understand. You're not a wave, you're part of the ocean.'"*   —*Morrie Schwartz, Professor and Lou Gehrig's Disease Patient*

---

*From Albom, M. (1997). *Tuesdays with Morrie.* New York: Doubleday, pp. 179–180.

OTHER PERSPECTIVES

Teamwork Requires Empowerment

"Teamwork requires empowerment, a willingness and commitment to 'let go' of self (one's own ideas, plans, strategies) to the benefit of the group. As I see it, there are five stages of empowerment:

"1. Letting go of self-promotion
"2. Believing that others are capable and competent
"3. Trusting others
"4. Willingness to forgo one's own processes/plans/strategies to give others a chance
"5. Sharing the outcomes/celebrating success"

—Sylvia Whiting, PhD, RN, CS

Related Skills: Developing Empowered Partnerships, Managing Conflict Constructively.

Critical Thinking Exercises

1. In a group, in a personal journal, or both:
    a. Think about a group you currently belong to (e.g., your peers, colleagues, or another group) in relation to the stages of team building shown in Box 6–7 (page 222). What stage is your group in?
    b. Share your best and worst experience with being part of a team. Consider what went right and why you think it went right and what went wrong and why you think it went wrong.
2. Practice brainstorming as a group. Get in a group of six to ten persons. Name one person the recorder and have him use a flip chart or black board. Identify a problem you'd like to resolve or a situation that could be improved (e.g., how you could get teenagers to come to a meeting on sex education). For 30 minutes, have group members each share ideas to be recorded by the recorder without interpretation. Once you're finished, spend 10 minutes discussing what happened (the group dynamics) as you brainstormed.
3. Determine whether you can achieve the learning outcomes at the beginning of this skill.

References

Carver, I. (1996). The six elements of team building. *Nursing Spectrum (FL Ed), 6*(3), 5.
Glaser, R., Glaser, C. (1994). *Building a winning team.* King of Prussia, PA: Organization Design and Development.

Paul, S. (1998). The advanced practice/staff nurse partnership: Building a winning team. *Critical Care Nurse, 18*(2), 92–97.

Porter-O'Grady, T., Wilson, C. (1999). *The healthcare teambook.* St. Louis: Mosby.

Pritchett, P. (1994). *The team member handbook for teamwork.* Dallas, TX: Pritchett and Associates.

9. USING INFORMATION EFFECTIVELY

Definition

Knowing how to find, interpret, and apply information.

Learning Outcomes

After you study this section and complete the accompanying exercises you should be able to:

- Identify ways to keep your files or notes more organized and easy to use.
- Demonstrate the ability to access and apply information.
- Explain how to prioritize information.

Thinking Critically about Using Information

As the amount of information in the world explodes, knowing how to *find, interpret,* and *use* information is as important as knowing how to *memorize* information. You can't carry around everything in your head. In many situations, you'll need to access and use information independently. Whether you're getting information from a book, a journal, a professional, or the Internet, it's important to determine whether the information is accurate, reliable, and applicable to the situation at hand.

Strategies for Using Information Effectively

1. **Learn how to use library resources:** Indexes, catalogs, interlibrary loan services, circulation department, reference department, audiovisual services, and computer searches (Table 6–4).

TABLE 6–4	What's Covered by Different Computer Databases*
COMPUTER DATABASES	**WHAT'S COVERED**
CINAHL (Cumulative Index to Nursing and Allied Health Literature)	Over 300 English language nursing journals, plus primary journals from allied health.
MEDLINE (Medical Literature Analysis and Retrieval System Online)	Most comprehensive online resource for national and international medical literature.
CHID (Combined Health Information Database)	Almost 50,000 citations and abstracts of information for health professionals, patients, and the general public.
HLTH (Health Planning and Administration)	Management, health care planning, organization, financing, manpower, patient education, accreditation, and other related subjects.
CATLINE (Catalog Online)	Over 500,000 references for books and serials cataloged at the National Library of Medicine.
HAPI (Health and Psychological Instruments Online)	Documents published in English for researchers, administrators, educators, and practitioners in health fields and the behavioral and psychological science.
AVLINE (Audiovisual Catalog Online)	Includes over 11,000 audiovisual packages covering a broad range of health-related subjects.
BIOETHICSLINE	Citations dealing with ethical questions arising in health care or biomedical research.
CANR (CANCERLIT)	All aspects of cancer from 1963 to present, updated monthly.

*Data from Burns, N., Groves, S. (1997). *The practice of nursing research: Conduct, critique, and utilization* (3rd ed.). Philadelphia: W.B. Saunders, pp. 126–128.

2. **Search the Internet as well as the preceding sources.** The preceding may not retrieve the most current, relevant, and useful information.
3. **Determine whether the sources are reliable.**
   - Can they be considered authorities on the subject?
   - What are their educational backgrounds and credentials?
   - What references are they using?
     - Are they up-to-date?

- Are journals peer reviewed or refereed?*
- Are publishers reputable?

- Do they have a vested interest (e.g., if drug information is being provided, is the drug company paying them?).

4. **Decide whether the information is applicable** in the context of the current situation (e.g., is the information relevant to your client(s)' sex, age, culture, developmental stage, socioeconomic factors?).

5. **If the information is questionable,** compare it with at least two other reputable sources.

6. **When you read information in newspapers or nonprofessional magazines,** verify it by checking original sources. Watch for follow-up articles and read letters to the editor (often you find thoughtful and professional commentary there).

7. **When overwhelmed, ask for help.** Librarians, nurse educators, pharmacists, and other professionals can point you in the right direction.

8. **Develop information management skills** so that you can access the most important information quickly.

- Find a way to keep what you really need in the forefront and what you *might* need in background files. For example, when I read an article, I make a document with the bibliographic citation and key points on my computer. Then I put the actual articles in a file cabinet in case I need to look into more detail later.
- Take notes or draw mind maps (see page 273) as you read. Revise them at least once to force yourself to do more in-depth thinking about what's most important.
- Get rid of irrelevant or unimportant information.
- Organize related information into separate files or clusters that are easily accessible. For example, I put articles together according to their relevance to topics or book chapters.
- Put the information on the computer whenever possible.

9. **Carry a little notebook or make yourself a cheat sheet** with key information that you need (e.g., formulas, lab values).

---

*This information can be found in the front of the journal, usually where you find journal information like address and listing of editorial board members.

OTHER PERSPECTIVES

Information Explosion? Yeah, right.

Duh and yeah right have arisen to fill a void in the language. . . . Fewer questions these days can effectively be answered with yes or no. . . . The information age . . . is more complicated than yes or no. It's more subtle . . . more loaded with content and hype and media manipulation than [in] my childhood.   —Courtesy of *The New York Times*

CRITICAL MOMENTS

Turning Information into Knowledge

You can't equate *information* with *knowledge*. Information is simply a group of facts. Turn information into knowledge by analyzing the data, identifying patterns and relationships, and working to gain insight into what the information implies.

Use Your Noodle as Well as Your Computer

Computerized information is only as good as the mind that interprets it. Computers aren't able to *think;* they have no common sense; and they "believe" anything anyone tells them. In fact, computers simply shuffle data around like books on a tabletop. It's up to you to discriminate and decide which "books" apply and whether they are the latest "copyright."

Use your noodle (brain) to interpret the information *in context* of each situation. Ask questions like, *How does this information apply to this particular case? How can I be sure this information is up to date?* And, *Does this sound reasonable?*

Critical Thinking Exercises

1. In a group, exchange information management problems and strategies you've found helpful. Choose three strategies you can use.
2. Together with one or two peers, pick a topic you'd like to know more about. Then using the library and the Internet and sharing what you found, choose 10 relevant articles on the topic.
   - Narrow the articles down to the two that are the most relevant and usable.
   - Explain how you will use the information.
3. Draw a mind map showing the relationships between the most important information presented in this section.
4. Determine whether you can achieve the learning outcomes at the beginning of this skill.

References

Burns, N., Groves, S. (1997). *The practice of nursing research: Conduct, critique, and utilization* (3rd ed.). Philadelphia: W.B. Saunders.

Johnson, M., Reineck, C., Daigle-Bjerke, et al. (1995). Understanding research articles. *Journal of Nursing Staff Development, 1*(2), 95–99.

Polit, D., Hungler, B. (1999). *Nursing research* (6th ed.). Philadelphia: Lippincott–Williams & Wilkins.

Sparks, S. (1998). World Wide Web search tools. *Image: Journal of Nursing Scholarship, 30*(2), 167–171.

10. OUTCOME-FOCUSED WRITING (WRITING WITH A PURPOSE)

Definition

Knowing how to change content and style of writing depending on what you aim to do.

Learning Outcomes

After you study this information and complete the accompanying exercises you should be able to:

- Improve the clarity of your writing by using specific strategies.
- Evaluate your writings to determine if they meet your intended purpose.
- Express the value of collaborating to improve writing projects.

Thinking Critically about Writing

Many of us don't feel like we're getting anything done unless our pens or fingers are moving and we're actually beginning to see the final form of our paper. However, from writing nurses' notes to writing formal papers, the time you take to clearly identify *what* you aim to do and *how* you can best do it is crucial to getting the final product you want. Writing, like any other skill, takes practice. The more you do it in the context of different situations—whether it be writing on the job or writing for school or publication—the better you become.

Strategies for Outcome-focused Writing

1. Determine exactly *what* you aim to do.*
   - Communicate (inform, instruct, or persuade)?
     Examples: Essays, term papers, articles, memos, letters, charting.
   - Form values (clarify your own values or explain them to others)?
     Examples: Personal journals, essays, term papers, articles, letters.
   - To learn (sort out and remember thoughts about specific topics rather than communicate)?
     Examples: Personal journals, note taking.
2. Decide exactly *who* will read your writing and keep this in mind as you write. Change your style accordingly. *Examples:* You write things differently:
   - If your boss or instructor is going to read it than if you were writing for a friend.
   - If your audience is lay people who don't know medical terms than if you're writing for nurses.
3. Identify what *content* you need to include to achieve your purpose.
   - What exactly are you writing *about*?
   - Make an outline, jot down topic headings, or draw a mind map (see page 273).
4. Decide what *type* of writing will best achieve your purpose.*
   - **Expressive:** *This is what I see, think, and feel.*
   - **Persuasive:** *This is what I believe, and this is why you should believe it.*
   - **Narrative:** *This is what happened (what I observed and heard) and then. . . .*
   - **Informational:** *This is what I know and how I know it. This is what others know and how I know they know it.*
5. Identify one to four outcomes you hope to achieve (this depends on length of the paper).
   Example Outcome: My teacher will read a paper that explains my beliefs on prolonging life in terminal illness and follows the guidelines given in the assignment.
6. Use headings to let the reader know what's coming up (see the headings throughout this book).

---

*You may have more than one purpose in one paper.

- Keep paragraphs short and focused on one idea at a time. Once you've written the paragraphs, evaluate how they relate to the headings you've used.
  - Have you wandered from the topic?
  - Do you need to change the heading?
  - Can you make the headings more interesting?
7. Keep it simple: simple terms make it easier to understand.
8. When you find yourself struggling with long sentences or paragraphs, consider whether bullets or numbered points could express the information more easily.
   - See how easy it is to read these short points?
   - Our brains do better with short phrases or sentences than long ones.
   - Bulleted points are actually also easier to write.
9. Use:
   - Examples and analogies to make your point and show why your information is relevant.
   - Tables and illustrations to increase understanding.
   - Active voice (e.g., "people see different things" rather than "different things are seen by people") and action verbs (e.g., "turn the patient" rather than "the patient is turned") to engage the reader.
10. Develop your own style. Don't be afraid to let your personality come through rather than sticking to strict, formal rules (check style requirements first if you're writing a formal paper, a school paper, or for a journal, see Box 6–8, page 232).
11. Give yourself enough time to write at least two drafts. Critically evaluate your first and final draft (see Box 6–9, page 235).
12. Got writers' block? See Box 6–10, page 235.

 CRITICAL MOMENTS

Writing Helps You Think

Once I asked a nurse if he wished he could do his charting by just dictating to a tape recorder. He responded, "Not really. When I write, I think." Then I asked, "What if you could dictate, then print out your notes and read them?" He responded, "Maybe then I'd like it because I could still evaluate my thoughts and see what I missed." When charting, evaluate your thinking—look for flaws and correct them. When thinking about something important, put your thoughts down on paper. It helps you stay focused and *evaluate* thoughts as you write.

Text continued on page 236

| BOX 6–8 | **Ten Strategies for School Papers** |

1. **Give yourself enough time** to complete the following steps:
   Plan: Determine your purpose and theme and set a schedule.
   Write: Write your paper according to the plan (you may, however, change the plan
   somewhat as you write if necessary; the point is to start with some sort of plan).
   Revise: Evaluate and improve (get others' input if possible).
   Edit: Proofread and correct.
2. **Before starting the assignment,** carefully review your instructor's requirements, including
   style requirements (formal, informal, type of citations, etc.). Make a checklist of what's most
   important to do. Keep the checklist in a place where you readily see it (e.g., at the front of
   your notebook or beginning of your computer file for the paper). Refer to the checklist
   frequently to make sure you're focusing your paper in such a way that it meets the most
   important criteria being graded.
   Example checklist:
   ☐ 25% of grade is on description of nursing theory.
   ☐ 50% of grade is on analysis and application of nursing theory.
   ☐ 25% of grade is on format (grammar, spelling, bibliography).
   ☐ Make sure to focus on how the theory can be applied *today.*
   ☐ Wants lots of examples.
3. **Start by discovering your thoughts and ideas** without being concerned about grammar or
   spelling.
   • List key ideas and questions that come to mind. Then review your ideas and ask yourself,
     What questions or thoughts do these ideas raise? Write these questions and thoughts
     down too.
   • Share your thoughts, feelings, and perceptions with friends. Ask them what questions or
     thoughts are raised for *them.*
   • If you express yourself well orally, put your thoughts on a tape recorder; then take notes
     on new ideas as you listen to yourself.
   • Keep a running list of your own ideas and ideas from your readings (be sure to cite your
     references in your notes or you might forget where the information came from and be
     accused of plagiarism).
   • Do your bibliography as you go along. When you encounter an interesting reference,
     immediately write down the full citation.
   • Think about using mind mapping (see pages 272 to 274).
4. **Develop one central idea, issue, or theme** that you can explain to someone in two or three
   sentences.
5. **Make an outline or simply list headings** of things you want to cover. Once you've listed
   your headings, number them in order of importance; then decide a logical flow of headings.

BOX 6–8	**Ten Strategies for School Papers** *Continued*

6. **Write the first draft in as concentrated a time as possible,** with as few interruptions as possible. Be realistic—this doesn't mean pulling an all-nighter.

7. **As you write, visualize your instructor** in your mind's eye: Predict what he or she will want to know and provide the information. If you don't want to visualize your instructor, visualize someone else you know who is inquisitive.

8. **Remember the Three T's.**
Tell them what you're going to tell them (introduction).
Tell them (body).
Tell them what you told them (summary).

9. **Once you've written the first draft, revise and improve,** preferably a few days later to give yourself a fresh eye. **Revising is as important as writing a first draft:** This is when you apply critical thinking to your own work and challenge yourself to write (and think) more clearly. Revising entails asking yourself questions like:

   • How well is the central idea of the paper addressed *early* in the paper? Somewhere early in the paper you should have something like, The purpose of this paper is . . . or This paper addresses . . . . (use these exact words). It won't be unusual to find a strong statement of this sort buried in the middle of your first draft (probably because your mind was on a roll at that point) or at the end, when you were making your final statements. Move these statements to the introduction.

   • How does my paper compare with my initial checklist of key points (see No. 2 above)?

   • How persuasively have I made my points or explained why I've come to the conclusions I've presented? (For example, writing, I've struggled with these issues and have decided . . . because. . . .)

   • How clearly does my summary describe what the paper addressed?

   • How can I make the introduction and summary catchy or inspiring?

Box continued on following page

BOX 6–8	**Ten Strategies for School Papers** *Continued*

10. **Edit your paper** to increase clarity and correct grammar and spelling problems.
    - Have someone else proofread your paper. You won't be able to proofread it well because you've looked at it too often and too long.
    - If you can't get someone else to proofread, READ YOUR PAPER OUT LOUD, or you'll miss important corrections. When you read silently, your brain edits without your realizing it. When you read your paper *out loud,* you'll *hear* your mistakes.
    - Trim the fat: Get rid of unnecessary words. Wordy sentences muddle your message and dilute its impact. For example, compare the clarity of the messages below (*b* says the same thing as *a,* only extra words are eliminated).
        a. *Altogether too many students feel that writing should be taught only to those people who want to go into journalism once they have finished school. What these students don't realize is that their efforts in practicing writing can greatly enhance their general ability to think critically.*
        b. *Many students feel that writing should be taught only to those who want to go into journalism. What these students don't realize is that practicing writing can enhance critical thinking.*
    - Play ICM (**I C**aught **M**e): Check yourself for repetition. We tend to use the same words over and over, making them lose their impact. Sometimes we even write two sentences back to back that essentially say the same thing. Compare the clarity of *a* and *b* below. I played ICM with *a* to get *b.*
        a. *When thinking about how to write, think about what's most important. If you focus your thinking on what's most important, you'll improve your thinking and your grades.*
        b. *When writing, stay focused on what's most important. You'll clarify your thoughts and improve your grades.*
      In *a* I recognized there were too many "think's" and "thinking's" and found ways of getting rid of them.
    - If using a computer, run a grammar check.

| BOX 6–9 | **Critically Evaluating Important Essays, Papers, Letters,* and Memos*** |

Using the guide below, rate how satisfied you are with *what* you wrote and *how* you wrote it on a 1–10 scale (10 = very satisfied with your product, and 1 = not at all satisfied).

____ It gives a good first impression of my work.*

____ The main purpose or objective is clearly stated at the beginning of the paper.*

____ Major headings are listed, and the paragraphs pertain to the headings.*

____ The paper shows that I followed instructions for *content* and *format* carefully (compare paper with assignment).

____ The paper is written specifically for whom I expect to read it.*

____ Opinions given are supported by facts.*

____ If I pull out all the headings and list them on a piece of paper, they show logical progression.*

____ I checked spelling.*

____ I asked someone to critique my first draft.*

____ I asked someone to proofread my final draft.*

____ Overall, based on the above, I'm pleased with this work.*

*The criteria can be applied to letters and memos as well as papers.

| BOX 6–10 | **Strategies for Getting Over Writer's Block** |

1. **Just get started,** letting your ideas flow onto the paper (or the computer) in whatever order they come to you. Sometimes, writing is like exercising. You need a warm-up period.
2. **Break the paper down into small tasks.** For example, if you can't seem to get started on the introduction, go on to address some of your other headings. It's not unusual to write the best introduction *after* you complete your paper. Doing easier headings before the introduction reduces your anxiety, helps you see progress, and gets your brain in "writing gear."
3. **Talk through your paper.** Call a friend and say, "I'm stuck on a point for my paper. Can you listen so I can explain it to you?" Write down key points as you explain them.

CRITICAL MOMENT

Watch Those Faxes, Emails, and Memos!

It's easy to become impulsive with emails, faxes, and interdepartmental memos. They are so quick that you want to just send them right off before you've given them the thought and attention they need. Think about whether you need to take the time to critically evaluate what you've written.

Also remember that faxes, emails, and memos may be subject to more eyes than you intend. Be careful with what you write and how you say it. If you want to be assured of privacy, send it regular mail and mark it private.

OTHER PERSPECTIVES

Sweating Our Writers' Block

Once I asked someone, "Do you know how to get rid of writers' block?" He replied, "Yeah. You sit in front of the computer and stare at the blank screen until beads of sweat form on your forehead and you sweat it out."

Critical Thinking Exercises

1. Pair off with a partner and exchange brainstorming lists.
   - Each of you add to the other person's list of ideas.
   - Then switch them back and have the original author circle three or four ideas that are closely related, including what the partner added.
   - As partners, write one or two sentences connecting the ideas.
2. Pick a controversial issue and a partner.
   a. One of you write a short pro paper, and the other a short con paper.
   b. Then switch papers and edit and improve each other's papers, keeping in mind the original purpose of the paper.
3. Keep your papers in a portfolio.
   a. Ask if you can improve or revise one of them to meet a course objective. Hand in both the old and new papers.
   b. Evaluate them according to the criteria in the checklist in Box 6–9.
4. Offer to critique and proofread peers' papers. It's great practice for writing.
5. Keep a journal. Practice letting your thoughts flow.

References

Brown, H., Sorrell, J. (1993). Use of clinical journals to enhance critical thinking. *Nurse Educator, 18*(5), 16–18.

Lashley, M., Wittstadt, R. (1993). Writing across the curriculum: An integrated curricular approach to developing critical thinking through writing. *Journal of Nursing Education, 32*(9), 422–424.

Paul, R. (1993). *Critical thinking: How to prepare students for a rapidly changing world.* Santa Rosa, CA: Foundation for Critical Thinking.

Ruggiero, V. (1988). *Teaching thinking across the curriculum.* New York: Harper & Row.

Ruggiero, V. (1991). *The art of thinking: A guide to critical and creative thought* (3rd ed.). New York: HarperCollins.

Response Key

Because the practice exercises are *open ended,* the following are **example responses** for the practice exercises, not the **only responses.** If you have questions about whether your responses are appropriate, check with your instructor. If a number isn't listed below, it's because giving an example response is inappropriate for that particular exercise.

CHAPTER 1

Example Responses for Critical Thinking Exercises (pages 20 and 21)

4. Self-centered people may focus too much on the results *they* want, rather than understanding that asking the question, What exactly are the results you want? means that you must think about the desired results in terms of the key players involved. For example, if you're working on a committee, to think critically you need to focus on the desired results from the group's perspective, rather than only your own.

5. (a) Facts are clearly observable and easily validated to be true. Opinions may vary depending on personal perspectives: they may or may not be valid. (b) The best way to determine if an opinion is valid is to ask for the facts or evidence that supports the opinion.

8. (a) Paraphrase any of the definitions beginning on page 8. (b) *Thinking* is basically *any mental activity*—it can be aimless

and uncontrolled. Critical thinking is controlled, purposeful, and more likely to lead to obvious beneficial results. (c) Four reasons are listed on pages 4–6. (d) Critical thinking focuses on achieving outcomes (results). (e) Your answer should be based on comparing yourself to the characteristics, traits, and dispositions found on pages 11–13. (f) Both critical thinking and problem solving focus on finding effective solutions. Critical thinking requires a more *proactive* approach, focusing on predicting, preventing, detecting, and managing problems and on finding ways to improve things, even when they are satisfactory. (g) See page 15.

CHAPTER 2

Example Responses for Critical Thinking Exercises (pages 40–41)

2. Critical thinking is often enhanced by our ability to use resources and teach ourselves. If we know how to take advantage of our preferred learning styles, we'll learn more easily and efficiently.

4. (a) Feelings have a tremendous impact on *what and how* we think. Those of us who are driven by feelings are likely to have more problems thinking critically, especially when situations are emotionally charged. (b) Thinking critically requires that you *recognize* feelings and their im-

pact on thinking and then use your head to apply logical and ethical reasoning principles. All too often we aren't even aware of deep strong feelings involved in certain situations. Those of us who are able to connect with emotions and give them the attention they deserve—to make them explicit, to accept them, and recognize their influence over thinking—can facilitate more logical, sensible thinking.

5. **(b)** Once you're aware of your thinking style—your usual approaches to gaining understanding and making decisions—and get in touch with your talents and blind spots, you can find ways to improve. **(c)** Habits are automatic. We do them without thinking. When we have deeply ingrained habits such as the ones that inhibit critical thinking on pages 36–38, we may *believe* we're thinking critically but are blind to how our habits are inhibiting our reasoning. If we create new habits that promote critical thinking like Covey's habits on page 19, we'll be more likely to automatically think critically.

Example Responses for Critical Thinking Exercises (pages 54–55)

1. Sometimes the terms *goals* and *outcomes* are used interchangeably. However, it's more correct to use *goals* when stating general intent (what you aim to do) and to use *outcome* to clearly describe what you expect to accomplish from the perspectives of others (outcomes are *specific results* that will be observed when your goal is achieved). *Example goal:* I want to teach Mr. Molinas about diabetes. *Example outcome:* By 4 weeks, Mr. Molinas will be able to give his own insulin and state how he will manage his dosage based on

his diet, activity level, and glucose monitor readings.

3. In the first situation you'd encourage creative, off-the-top-of-your-head ideas, while in the second situation, because of the risks involved, you'd want sound, evidence-based ideas.

5. Jack and Jill are goldfish, and a cat knocked the fish tank on the floor, shattering it. You could have asked, Who are Jack and Jill?

6. **(a)** Critical thinking is purposeful, outcome-directed (results-oriented) thinking. If you aren't clear and specific about the expected outcomes, you're not thinking critically. **(b)** See critical thinking strategies on pages 46–48. **(c)** If we can't communicate effectively, gain trust, and establish good interpersonal relationships, we have difficulty getting the facts we need to think critically. **(d)** See Using Logic, Intuition, and Trial-and-Error, page 45. **(f)** See Figure 2–1, page 50.

CHAPTER 3

Example Responses for Critical Thinking Exercises (pages 70 and 71)

2. You need to be able to describe critical thinking and know what critical thinking skills entail before you can truly become a critical thinker. Learning by *doing* in simulated exercises, such as those in Chapter 5, can help you acquire and remember key knowledge and skills required for critical thinking.

4. *I don't know* isn't an acceptable answer. A critical thinker who is oriented to satisfying customers would respond, *I'll find out.* Finding out will help her broaden her knowledge and help Mr. Gimenez.

5. In the presence of known problems, you predict the *most likely* and *most dangerous* complications and take immediate action to (a) prevent them and (b) be prepared to manage them in case they can't be prevented. *Example:* If you're going to care for someone with a wired jaw and you aren't familiar with the care of someone with a wired jaw, you'd look it up so that you'd know common and dangerous complications (e.g., in this case, one dangerous complication is aspiration because the person is unable to open his mouth, so you would have wire cutters near by). You also look for evidence of *risk and causative* factors (things we know cause problems or put people at risk for problems). You then aim to control these factors to prevent the problems themselves. *Example:* In the case of the wired jaw, you'd assess for nausea (a risk factor for aspiration). If nausea was present, you'd ask for an antinausea drug, you'd hold food, and you'd keep suction equipment and wire cutters close by.

6. (b) See Goals of Nursing and Their Implications on page 60. (c) It means that (1) care is directed at reaching observable beneficial results *in the client,* (2) we identify expected outcomes based on the results we know are likely to be achieved according to data (or evidence) gathered in clinical studies, and (3) we choose treatment plans most likely to work based on evidence from clinical studies (we know which treatments work best for certain problems). (d) Both DT and PPM focus on treating problems. However, PPM is more proactive and focused on prevention through early intervention than the DT model is.

Example Responses for Critical Thinking Exercises (pages 93 and 94)

1. The terms *clinical judgment, clinical reasoning,* and *critical thinking* are often used interchangeably. You use clinical reasoning and critical thinking to make a clinical judgment.

2. Clinical judgment often requires thinking on your feet. It also requires knowing when to take your time and contact experts before making a decision. Clinical judgment entails things like knowing what to look for, how to recognize when a patient's status is changing, and what to do about it. It requires theoretical and experiential knowledge and application of standards, ethics, and principles of nursing process.

3. In today's competitive health care arena the organizations who succeed will be those who best satisfy their customers needs. We also realize that people deserve to be treated in a timely way by honest, courteous professionals.

4. You could irrigate a nasogastric tube if the facility permitted it, you've received permission from your instructor, you have the required knowledge and level of competence, the procedure is reasonable and prudent, and you're willing to assume accountability for how you perform the procedure and the patient response to the procedure.

5. (a) It's unlikely that the off-going nurse has really assessed the family's needs. It's highly unlikely that the family is doing fine. It appears as though the family has had limited involvement in the child's care. (b) You need to assess the family's needs and begin to include interventions that meet these needs in the nursing plan

(e.g., allow the family to spend more time with the child).

6. **(a)** See Rule (the terms *diagnose* and *diagnosis* have legal implications) on page 74. **(b)** Decision making is *guided by* ethics codes and national and facility standards and guidelines. **(c)** See Box 3–10, page 91, A Common Approach to Identifying Immediate Priorities. **(d)** Some suggestions: Write an outcome statement that clearly shows what you'll be able to do when you improve your ability to use good clinical judgment. Identify ways you can increase your theoretical and experiential knowledge. Get actively involved in seeking out learning resources and experiences. Make a commitment to study judiciously and prepare for learning experiences so that you can get the most out of them. Get involved in helping as a community, church, hospital, or nursing home volunteer. Seek out a mentor.

CHAPTER 4

Example Responses for Critical Thinking Exercises (pages 114 to 116)

Moral and Ethical Reasoning Exercises
1. Ask for a family meeting to make the decision, including an ethicist, trusted friends, or person from the clergy to help.
2. Justice, beneficence, accountability.

Nursing Research Exercises
1. **(b)** Get the actual article. Check whether it comes from a refereed journal. Get more articles on the same topic. Check with a research text or find an article addressing how to analyze research studies. Discuss the results with experts and peers.

3. **(b)** These articles are more likely to be reliable.

Example Responses for Critical Thinking Exercises (page 129)

Teaching Others, Teaching Ourselves, Test Taking
1. A major nursing goal is to promote independence and optimum functioning. By teaching people about their health care, we empower them to be independent and healthy.
4. **(b)** Knowing how to memorize efficiently helps you remember the facts you need to think critically (critical thinking requires knowledge). Reasoning, or thinking your way through learning, helps you master and remember information from your own perspective.

CHAPTER 5

Practice Exercises

1. Identifying Assumptions (pages 137 to 139)
1. There's not enough evidence to indicate that the patient needs instruction. Many people are fully knowledgeable about their diet but aren't able to stick to it.
2. You might waste your time teaching information the patient already knows. You might alienate the patient: Who likes to be taught things they already know? The patient gets the message that you don't understand the problem—that you jump to conclusions.
3. *Scenario One.* **(a)** She seems to have assumed that she can *create* a positive attitude for Jeff by talking about advances in diabetic care. **(b)** She needed to assess Jeff's *human response* to learning he's a diabetic. Jeff may be well aware of advances

in diabetic care but is still having trouble coming to terms with having to regulate his diet and take insulin for the rest of his life. She didn't *assess* before *acting*. **(c)** Jeff probably thinks Anita is a know-it-all because she didn't take the time to find out what his point of view on the situation was. It's a real turn-off when someone starts trying to change your attitude before he or she finds out what your attitude *is*.

Scenario Two. **(a)** She seems to have assumed the mother can read and that the mother will let her know if she has questions. **(b)** If the mother can't read or is embarrassed to ask questions, the child may have inadequate care from his mother. If harm results from the nurse's failure to determine the mother's understanding, the nurse may be accused of negligence.

Scenario Three. **(a)** That he would have the *desired* response to the drug without any adverse reactions. **(b)** It's likely that she was concerned that Mr. Schmidt wouldn't respond to the diuretic as expected—that he might experience an adverse reaction. **(c)** She probably thought the physician wouldn't like it if she challenged his judgment.

2. Identifying an Organized and Comprehensive Approach to Discovery (Assessment)
(pages 141 to 143)
1. The body systems approach to assessment (Fig. 3–3, page 80) is probably the best method. Or you may choose the head-to-toe approach, clustering signs and symptoms of medical problems after you perform the assessment.
2. A nursing model approach. Boxes 3–5 and 3–6 (pages 80 and 81) show examples of nursing models.

3. *Scenario One.* **(a)** Assess the extent of Pearl's voluntary movement (can she wiggle her toes?); color of toes and skin around cast edges; whether Pearl feels numbness or tingling in her foot or leg; whether there is any edema of the leg or toes; the quality of the dorsalis pedis pulse; whether Pearl perceives a needle prick as being sharp; whether her toes are warm or cool. **(b)** Assessing each of the above helps you detect *early* signs of circulatory problems, nerve compression, or skin irritation: If you find one area that begins to exhibit abnormal assessment findings (e.g., edema), you should increase the frequency and intensity of assessment of *other* areas (e.g, skin color). Specific relevance of each area of assessment follows: Checking movement, numbness, and sensation monitors for nerve compression. Checking for color, edema, pulse quality, warmth monitors circulation and skin condition. **(c)** Check circulation by assessing the dorsalis pedis pulse quality and capillary refill in toes; check for nerve compression by asking her to wiggle her toes and ask whether there is any numbness or tingling. If these are satisfactory, you might choose to put a warm sock over the toes; encourage her to wiggle her toes frequently to increase the circulation, and continue to monitor her dorsalis pedis pulse, toe temperature, and toe sensation closely.

Scenario Two. **(a)** You'd look up digoxin in a reference; then assess as follows. *To assess for therapeutic effect*, check to see if Mr. Wu's serum digoxin level is within therapeutic range (0.8–2 ng/ml). Determine status of cardiac symptoms, as compared with baseline (status of apical/radial pulse rate and rhythm, lung sounds, urine output, edema, activity tolerance). *To assess for adverse reactions,* check Mr. Wu for signs and symptoms of any of the adverse reactions listed in the drug reference. You'd also assess for contraindications and toxicity/overdose, as follows. *To assess for contraindications,* check Mr. Wu for signs and symptoms of any of the contraindications listed in the drug reference. Most common contraindications for digoxin include serum potassium levels <3.5 mEq/L (increases the risk of toxicity); pulse rate less than 60 or physician-prescribed parameters; clinical signs of toxicity/overdose. *To assess for toxicity/overdose,* check Mr. Wu for signs and symptoms of toxicity/overdose. Most common signs and symptoms of digoxin toxicity include serum digoxin level >2 ng/ml; atrioventricular block (PR interval >0.24 sec); progressive bradycardia, nausea, vomiting, visual disturbances (blurring, snowflakes, yellow-green halos around images). **(b)** If no *therapeutic effect* is achieved by giving a drug or if the person is experiencing *adverse reactions,* you need to question whether there needs to be a change in dosage or whether the drug should be continued at all. If you identify contraindications to giving the drug, you need to withhold the drug. If you identify signs of toxicity/overdose, it's especially important to withhold the drug because you'd be *adding* to the toxicity/overdose problem.

Scenario Three. **(a)** *Vital signs:* Take temperature, pulse, respirations, and blood pressure. *Eye opening:* Call Gerome's name. Tell him to open his eyes. If no response, pinch him. *Best motor response:*

Ask him to move each extremity. Use a pin prick or pinch him and see if he can tell you where he feels it. If no response, pinch him and note whether he flexes his extremity to withdraw from pain, flexes in spasm, or extends his extremity. *Best verbal response:* Ask him what his name is, where he is, and what day it is. Pupillary reaction: Determine size of each pupil in millimeters before flashing a light into it. Then flash a light into *each* pupil and observe whether it constricts briskly. *Purposeful limb movement:* Check each extremity by asking Gerome to move it, observing for muscle contraction (attempts to move), ability to lift extremity, and ability to lift extremity even though you try to hold it down. *Limb sensation:* Prick each limb with a sterile needle and ask Gerome what he feels (this may be unnecessary for Gerome, since he has a head injury rather than a spinal cord injury). *Seizure activity:* Observe for muscle twitching. *Gag reflex:* Place a clean tongue blade in the back of Gerome's throat and see if it triggers gagging. **(b)** By assessing all of these parameters, signs and symptoms of increased intracranial pressure can be detected early. Signs and symptoms of increased intracranial pressure are decreasing level of consciousness, increasing restlessness, irritability and confusion, stronger headache, nausea and vomiting, increasing speech problems, pupillary changes (dilated and nonreactive or constricted and nonreactive pupils), cranial nerve dysfunction, increasing muscle weakness, flaccidity, or coordination problems; seizures; decerebrate posturing (muscles stiff and extended, head retracted) and decorticate posturing (muscles rigid and still, with arms flexed, fists clenched, and legs extended)—these are both *late* signs of increased intracranial pressure. **(c)** Monitor *other* parameters of neurologic assessment closely for *other* signs of increased intracranial pressure. If there are no *other* changes and you can indeed arouse Gerome, you don't need to be immediately concerned; however, you should increase the frequency of assessment of all parameters until you're comfortable that the increased somnolence is merely a sign of the combined effects of fatigue and *existing* brain swelling (rather than increasing brain swelling). If you have ANY QUESTIONS about how to proceed, report the increased somnolence to your supervisor. **(d)** Check other neurologic parameters closely and report and record findings immediately; increase the frequency of assessment. **(e)** If the baseline pulse was rapid, this may be a normal finding. However, you should closely assess all the other assessment parameters to check for other reportable signs and symptoms. If the pulse is dropping to 60 beats per minute, closely monitor all the other assessment parameters and report the findings *immediately* (may be a sign of life-threatening increase in intracranial pressure).

3. Checking Accuracy and Reliability of Data (Validation) (page 150)

1. Talk with Mrs. Molinas and explore her feelings and concerns.
2. You may be able to turn on his blood glucose monitor and check it (some monitors automatically show the previous blood glucose level. If not, you can ask Mr. Nola to take it again now (quietly observe his technique). If he is proficient at performing a check for blood glucose, it's likely his previous result was correct. If the second reading is significantly different from the previous reading, consider whether there is a relationship between the change in blood sugar reading and recent food intake or peak insulin levels. I would consider the blood sugar reading the patient took with you observing as being most valid.
3. Take it in the right arm. Take it again in 15 minutes.
4. Explore with Mr. McGwire why he thinks he got his foot ulcers. Ask him to tell you what he does to avoid getting foot ulcers. He may be very knowledgeable about diabetic care and foot ulcers and still be getting these ulcers.

4. Distinguishing Normal from Abnormal/Identifying Signs and Symptoms (page 152)

1. **(a)** If you assumed this was an oral temperature, you should have "S" here. You may have placed a question mark here, which is actually a more correct response. You need to ask, *How was this temperature taken (orally? rectally? tympanic?).* **(b)** If you assumed the patient never has rales, you should have an "S" here. You may have placed a question mark here, which is actually a more correct response. You need to ask questions like, *What do the patient's lungs sound like when he's in his usual state of health? What is the respiratory rate? How far up the back can you hear the rales? Are there just a few rales or copious rales? When the patient coughs, do the rales clear?* **(c)** You may have put an "S" here, but *you really need to ask if this is a normal pattern for the person and why the person only sleeps*

3 hours at a time (e.g., it's not unusual for mothers of newborns to sleep only 3 hours at a time because of feeding schedules). **(d)** S. **(e)** O or question mark. This is usually a normal finding, but you may have placed a question mark because you wanted to know such things as *whether there's any drainage, whether the area is hot to touch, and whether the patient is afebrile.* **(f)** O. This is normal for a 2-year-old. **(g)** S. **(h)** You may have placed an "S" here, but a better response is a question mark. You need to ask, *What are the bathing practices of a person of this culture?* **(i)** S. This is likely to be a normal finding, since the dialysis takes over the work of the kidney. **(j)** S or question mark. The pulse is somewhat slow but might be normal for someone who is young and athletic or older and on cardiac medication. You may have wanted to ask, *What is this person's normal pulse?* or *Is the person taking any cardiac medications that slow the heart rate?*

2. The italicized words in the answers to number 1 provide examples of what else you might have wanted to know.

5. Making Inferences (Drawing Valid Conclusions) (pages 153 and 154)

1. I suspect this information indicates infection of some sort.
2. I suspect this information indicates financial problems.
3. I suspect this information indicates that the patient has trouble sticking to his diet.
4. I suspect this information indicates that the child wants to be sure his mother approves of his answer, or perhaps he is afraid.
5. I suspect this information indicates there is some medical reason for the grandmother's confusion.

6. Clustering Related Cues (Data) (page 155)

Scenario One. **(a)** Stung by a bee on the ear an hour ago; ear has no stinger, is red and swollen; no rash or wheezing; normal pulse and respirations. **(b)** Afraid he might die; wants to have a popsicle and watch TV. **(c)** Didn't make sure she had parents' phone number down (investigate whether this was lack of knowledge or oversight); doesn't know first aid for a bee sting.

Scenario Two. **(a)** 41 years old; acute abdominal pain; vomiting for 2 days and unable to keep any food down; abdomen distended; no bowel sounds; scheduled to go to the operating room at 2 PM; pain suddenly getting worse; vital signs unchanged, except pulse is increased by approximately 30 beats/min. **(b)** 41-year-old businessman; hates everything about hospitals; scheduled to go to the operating room at 2 PM; worried because his brother died in the hospital after a car accident; suddenly experiencing *severe* pain.

7. Distinguishing Relevant from Irrelevant (pages 157 and 158)

Scenario One. **(a)** May be relevant because buspirone hydrochloride can cause confusion in the elderly. **(b)** May be relevant because it may be a sign of infection, which can cause confusion in the elderly. **(c)** May be relevant because it's indicative of previous cardiovascular disease, which is a risk factor for cerebrovascular accident (stroke), which may be the cause of the confusion. **(d)** May be relevant because dehydration in the elderly can cause electrolyte imbalance and confusion. **(e)** Not relevant. **(f)** Not relevant.

Scenario Two. **(a)** Probably relevant. It takes time to adjust to a diabetic regimen. **(b)**

Not relevant (not abnormal). (c) May be relevant (may feel constipation is caused by new diet). (d) May be relevant because she has to prepare meals for others, increasing temptation. (e) Very probably relevant. Someone who likes to cook usually takes joy in eating a variety of foods. (f) Relevant. She needs to eat even less than she will when her weight is within normal limits. (g) Not relevant (has nothing to do with sticking to a diabetic diet).

8. *Recognizing Inconsistencies (pages 159 and 160)*

Scenario One. (a) It doesn't make sense that she has only just started coming to prenatal clinic but has been going to birthing classes. If she hasn't had prenatal care until now, you wonder whether she's really happy about the baby coming or realizes the importance of prenatal visits. You may also wonder why her mother, rather than her boyfriend, came to the clinic visit. (b) Check her records to see if there's any mention of receiving prenatal care somewhere else for the earlier part of her pregnancy; ask her where she's been going to birthing classes; ask how her boyfriend and mother feel about the baby coming.

Scenario Two. Her age is inconsistent with risk factors for a myocardial infarction (MI). The *big picture* here—her age, absence of pain, and previously normal electrocardiogram—is inconsistent with the big picture of an MI. *Occasionally* people don't have pain when they have an MI, but usually there are other risk factors and signs and symptoms present. Her signs and symptoms are more consistent with those of a panic attack.

9. *Identifying Patterns (pages 161 and 162)*
   (a) Altered Respiratory Function. Signs and symptoms of respiratory function problems are present. (b) Normal Coping Pattern. There are no signs or symptoms of abnormal coping pattern. (c) Pattern of Potential (Risk) for Altered Bowel Elimination. There are risk factors for constipation but no signs and symptoms. (d) Normal Sleep-Rest Pattern. Considering the person works nights, there are no signs and symptoms of an abnormal sleep-rest pattern. (e) Potential (Risk) for Altered Sexual-Reproductive Pattern. There are risk factors for Altered Sexual-Reproductive Pattern.

10. *Identifying Missing Information (page 163)*
   (a) What are the person's *other* vital signs (pulse, blood pressure, temperature)? Is there a history of smoking? Is the person smoking now? How long has this pattern persisted? What does the person feel is contributing to this pattern? How does the person tolerate activity? (b) How does the husband feel about helping her? (c) Who is the major caregiver? What factors are contributing to the lack of roughage in his diet and his inadequate fluid intake? What's the patient's (or caregiver's) knowledge of how to prevent altered bowel elimination? Why does the patient spend most of his time in bed? How motivated is the patient to do the things necessary to prevent altered bowel elimination? (d) Does the person feel he's getting adequate rest? Are any sleeping aids being taken? If so, what are they? (e) What are the woman's feelings about having herpes? What does the woman know about herpes transmission? How does she feel

about telling prospective partners about the herpes? How does the patient plan to prevent herpes transmission?

11. Promoting Health by Identifying Risk Factors (page 165)

1. Do you have any family history of health problems? What's your ethnic background? Do you smoke? What do your usual meals consist of? Do you exercise regularly and get enough rest? How do you manage stress? Do you drink alcohol or take drugs that aren't prescribed? Are you sexually active? Do you wear your seat belt? What do you do to stay healthy?

2. Her age puts her at risk for osteoporosis. The history of falls together with the risk of osteoporosis put her at high risk for fractures. You need to look closely at why she is falling (e.g., balance problems? coordination problems? weakness or fatigue? vision problems? home hazards?). You should also assess calcium intake, which needs to be adequate to prevent osteoporosis.

3. Even though this is a social interaction, rather than professional nurse-patient interaction, keep in mind that because you're a nurse, he's likely to listen. Reenforce that he has a good question—that we all live longer now and that it's good to do things to increase the likelihood of living longer *and healthier*. Give some examples, like the importance of staying active and eating well. Stress the importance of annual exams that include blood studies to monitor things like cholesterol, blood sugar, and prostate specific antigen. Suggest doing this annual exam around a specific time (birthday, Christmas, etc.) so that he remembers.

12. Diagnosing Actual and Potential (Risk) Problems (page 169)

Scenario One. Potential for (or Risk for) Violence related to agitation and previous history of striking caregivers.

Scenario Two. Potential complications: hemorrhage, shock, vomiting with aspiration, pneumonia, infection, paralytic ileus.

Scenario Three. Hopelessness related to new diagnosis of terminal cancer as evidenced by statements of hopelessness and withdrawn behavior (sleeps most of the time, doesn't want to talk to anyone). *Powerlessness* is also an acceptable response. There is a fine line between these two diagnoses.

Scenario Four. History of smoking or lung disease, whether the fractures are stable (risk for punctured lung), whether he has pain that is preventing him from coughing and clearing his lungs (risk for pneumonia).

13. Setting Priorities (pages 171 to 173)

1. **(b)** (*a* is likely to be dealt with informally or at home. *c* will be covered by the diagnoses listed in *b*).

2. **Scenario One.** Reporting the chest pain should be your immediate priority. Myocardial infarction and pulmonary embolus, both serious problems, are potential complications of thrombophlebitis.

   Scenario Two. 1. **(a)** 3. **(b)** 2 or 3. **(c)** 2 or 3. 2. No response provided. 3. **(b)** This isn't a problem that *must* be addressed to achieve the major outcomes. It's unrealistic to try to resolve this problem in 2 days. Rather you'd be a good listener, provide support, and encourage him to seek support from family or counselors.

14. Determining Client-centered Expected Outcomes (page 176)

1. Client will maintain intact skin, free of signs of redness or irritation.
2. After suctioning, mouth, nose, and lungs will be clear.
3. After the health team conference the client will express feelings about powerlessness and relate increased sense of power over his situation as evidenced by statements that he is allowed to make as many choices about his own care as possible.
4. After irrigation, Foley catheter will be patent and draining urine.
5. Endotracheal tube will be out by (date).
6. Will demonstrate increased activity tolerance as evidenced by ability to walk the length of the hall and back by (date).

15. Determining Specific Interventions (pages 178 to 180)

1. **(a)** Monitor fluid intake every shift. Keep iced tea (patient's preference) at the bedside on ice. Encourage drinking at least 3 quarts during the day and 1 quart at night. Reinforce the importance of maintaining adequate hydration. Record fluid intake. **(b)** Monitor anxiety level. Encourage her to express feelings and concerns. Fully explain all procedures. **(c)** Monitor comfort level. After applying heat for 30 minutes, assist with range of motion exercises 3 times a day.
2. *Scenario.* **a.** **(1)** It's quite likely the children won't report finding ticks, increasing the likelihood that the mother won't know when the children may have been bitten. It also increases the likelihood that the ticks won't be properly disposed of. I doubt that there will be benefits from using this approach (punishment). **(2)**

It's possible that they may go looking for ticks, increasing the likelihood of being bitten. It's also possible that this approach might work, but the risks outweigh the benefits. **b.** Determine children's understanding of the severity of the consequences of tick bites and the importance of finding ways to avoid them. Initiate teaching as indicated. Explain to the children that they can best help by asking for insect repellent to be applied before going outside, reporting ticks found on themselves and on each other, and avoiding tall grass areas. Start a rule that the children can't go outside without first applying insect repellent. Have the mother praise good behavior (e.g., asking for insect repellent) verbally, rather than offering rewards. Instruct the mother not to offer rewards for finding ticks.

17. Determining a Comprehensive Plan/ Evaluating and Updating the Plan (pages 183 and 184)

1. **(a)** Not achieved. **(b)** Achieved. **(c)** Partially achieved; focus teaching toward mother's needs.
2. *Scenario. Discharge outcome:* Will be discharged home with husband able to demonstrate administration of epinephrine by 6/29. *Nursing diagnosis no. 1:* Knowledge Deficit (husband): Epinephrine administration. *Expected outcome:* Husband will relate knowledge of action and side effects of epinephrine and when to give epinephrine and demonstrate subcutaneous injection technique. *Interventions:* Provide husband with literature about epinephrine administration. Assess husband's knowledge of epinephrine action, side effects, and administration. Also

determine preferred learning style. Reinforce what he already knows; teach gaps in knowledge using the husband's preferred learning style. Record husband's progress toward expected outcome after each teaching session. *Nursing diagnosis no. 2:* Altered Comfort (itching feet) related to hives as evidenced by hives over feet. *Expected outcome:* Patient will experience decreased itching as evidenced by statements of increased comfort. *Interventions:* Assist patient to place feet in cool water prn. Medicate as ordered prn for itching. *Note:* You may have chosen another diagnosis, such as *Ineffective Coping,* for Mrs. Kooney, in the hope that you can help her cope with the possibility of learning how to give her own injections. However, in the interest of time, *teaching the husband* is first priority. **3.** You've identified a care variance and should seek multidisciplinary evaluation to determine whether additional treatment and resources are needed to improve outcomes. According to the predicted care, there should be no confusion. **4.** See Box 5–3, page 182.

Appendix A

Summary of What Some Experts Say about Critical Thinking

Richard Paul, author and director of research at the Center for Critical Thinking, describes critical thinking as thinking that's done under discipline and sound intellectual standards.[1] **To think critically you must:**

- Define your purpose and goals well
- Frame questions or problems precisely
- Carefully check information for its completeness and relevance
- Be able to trace implications and consequences
- Appreciate multiple perspectives and ways of looking at things
- Be disciplined, hold yourself to standards, and evaluate and correct your thinking

Paul addresses the need to develop what he calls intellectual traits, or habits of the mind, such as intellectual humility, integrity, courage, responsibility, and empathy (see Chapter 1, pages 10–11).

■ ■ ■

Stephen Brookfield, author and consultant, encourages us to gain control over our lives though critical evaluation of underlying beliefs and considering alternatives to those beliefs.[2] He views critical thinking as being:

- **Productive and positive.** Critical thinkers see themselves as creating and re-creating aspects of their personal, workplace, and political lives. They see the future as open and malleable rather than closed and fixed.
- **A process, not an outcome.** You can't be in a state of complete critical development.
- **Manifested in different ways, depending on the context in which it occurs.** The indicators of whether someone is thinking critically vary greatly: Sometimes the process is completely internal, and we can find evidence only in the person's writing or talking. Other times it can be evident through actions (people who renegotiate aspects of their work or relationships).
- **Triggered by positive as well as negative events.** Encountering negative events often causes us to question previously trusted assumptions. Encountering positive events—like falling in love or being unexpectedly successful at something—often causes us to inter-

[1]Paul, R. (1995). *Critical thinking: How to prepare students for a rapidly changing world.* Santa Rosa, CA: Foundation for Critical Thinking.

[2]Brookfield, S. (1987). *Developing critical thinkers.* San Francisco: Jossey-Bass.

pret our past actions and ideas from a new vantage point.

- **Emotive as well as rational.** Critical thinking isn't above the realm of feeling. Rather, emotions are central to the thinking process.

Brookfield addresses four components of critical thinking:

1. **Identifying and challenging assumptions:** Examining values, beliefs, rationales, and appropriateness of ideas that influence an action.
2. **Challenging the importance of context:** Examining the circumstances surrounding an action such as factors related to a patient's complaints or reaction to illness.
3. **Imagining and examining alternatives:** Generating new ideas and strategies and determining whether they're feasible.
4. **Reflective skepticism:** Questioning ideas that claim to be the answers for all problems.

■ ■ ■

Peter and Norene Facione are two researchers who have developed paper-and-pencil tests that they believe measure the ability and disposition to think critically. They view critical thinking as the "cognitive engine which drives problem-solving and decision-making."[3] The Faciones address the following elements of critical thinking:

- **Six critical thinking cognitive skills:** Interpretation, analysis, evaluation, inference, explanation, and self-regulation.[4]
- **Seven critical thinking dispositions, or habits of the mind:** Truthseeking, open-mindedness, analyticity, systematicity, critical thinking self-confidence, inquisitiveness, and maturity (see pages 12–13).[5]

■ ■ ■

Barbara K. Scheffer and Gaie Rubenfield, two nurse researchers at Eastern Michigan University, have conducted a Delphi study to define critical thinking in nursing based on input from various nursing experts, including myself. The study was completed in the summer of 1998 but was not published at the time of this book's publication. For more information, Scheffer and Rubenfield can be contacted at Eastern Michigan University, Department of Nursing, Ypsilanti, MI 48197.

---

[3]Facione, N., Facione, P., Sanchez, C. (1994). Critical thinking disposition as a measure of competent clinical judgment: The development of the California Critical Thinking Disposition Inventory. *Journal of Nursing Education, 33*(8), 345–351.

[4]Facione, P.A., Facione, N.C. (1992). *The California Critical Thinking Skills Test Manual.* Milbrae, CA: California Academic Press.

[5]Facione, P.A., Facione, N.C. (1992). *The California Critical Thinking Disposition Inventory (CCTD).* Milbrae, CA: California Academic Press.

RESOURCES FOR INFORMATION ON CRITICAL THINKING

Sonoma State University
The Center for Critical Thinking and Moral
  Critique
1801 E. Cotati Ave.
Rohnert Park, CA 94928
Phone: (707) 664-2940

Foundation for Critical Thinking
P.O. Box 302
Wye Mills, MD 21679
Phone: (800) 833-3645 or (410) 364-5082;
  fax: (410) 364-5215
Email: cct@sonoma.edu
Web site: http://www.sonoma.edu/cthink

California Academic Press
217 La Cruz Ave.
Millbrae, CA 94030
Phone: (650) 697-5628
Email: info@calpress.com
Web site: www.calpress.com

The National Center for Teaching Thinking
815 Washington St., Suite #8
Newtonville, MA 02160
Phone: (617) 965-4604; fax: (617) 965-4674
Email: rjscct@prodigy.net

What's Your Preferred Learning Style?

Overall Categories: Doer (kinesthetic), visual learner (observer, reader), auditory learner (listener)

Specific Categories: Logical learner, linguistic learner, spatial learner, musical learner

Almost everyone is a combination of two or more of these styles.

OVERALL CATEGORIES

Doers (Kinesthetic Learners)

Learn best by doing, moving, experiencing, or experimenting. For example, they'd rather play with a syringe and inject a dummy before reading the procedure.

Strategies to Take Advantage of Your "Doing" Style

1. Ask if you can start by *doing* (e.g., fiddling with equipment before reading about how to use it). Observing, reading, and listening will be more meaningful after you *do.*
2. Be sure you know the risks of doing first and find ways to minimize them (e.g., If you're playing on the computer, make sure you can't inadvertently erase a file).
3. When taking notes, use arrows to show relationships.
4. Pace up and down while reciting information to yourself.
5. Make tapes with the information you're trying to learn and play them while exercising (e.g., riding a bike), or read while riding a stationary bike.
6. Write key words in the air; use your fingers to help you remember (bend the forefinger as you memorize a concept, then the bend the next for the next concept, and so on).
7. Change positions frequently while studying; take frequent short breaks involving activity. This doesn't mean chatting with friends—it's too easy to get sidetracked.
8. Study in a rocking chair.
9. Study with background music.
10. Ask if you can do assignments in an active way (e.g., create a poster, be part of a discussion group).

Visual Learners

Learn best by watching first. For example, they'd rather *watch* someone give an injection before reading the procedure.

Strategies to Take Advantage of Your "Visual" Style

1. Ask to be included in observational experiences.
2. Sit in the front of the room, so you stay focused on the teacher, not on what's going on around you.
3. Take lots of notes and use a highlighter. Recopy your notes when you're studying.
4. In skills labs, don't go first. Rather, watch your classmates and take a later turn.
5. Read procedures through, focusing on illustrations.
6. Visualize procedures *in your mind's eye,* rather than trying to follow individual steps.
7. Write things down (e.g., things to be done, directions).
8. When learning new terms or concepts or trying to remember something, write them on "sticky notes" and put them where you'll see them frequently (the bathroom mirror, the computer).
9. Preview chapters by scanning headings and illustrations.

Auditory Learners
Learn best by hearing.

Strategies to Take Advantage of Your "Auditory" Style
1. Read by subvocalizing (mouth the words and almost whisper) and concentrate on hearing the words. This is especially important when reading test questions.
2. Just *listen* in class, focusing on hearing what the teacher *says* without taking notes; then make a copy of someone else's notes.
   - Tape classes and listen to the tapes two or three times before exams.
   - Ask if you can give an oral report or hand in an audio tape for extra credit.
   - Memorize by making up songs or rhymes.
   - Study with a friend, so you verbalize the information.
   - Tape yourself as you read key information out loud, then listen to the tapes.

SPECIFIC CATEGORIES

Logical Learners
Like to have things organized and consistent.

Strategies to Take Advantage of Your "Logical" Style
1. Recognize that organization and logical flow of content may be unique to each person: The way you might organize information might not be how someone *else* might organize it, even though both ways are useful.
2. When reading texts, jot down headings on separate pieces of paper, then write notes under the appropriate heading as you encounter information that belongs there. This way the chapter will be organized how *you* want it to be.

3. Organize and reorganize your notes.
4. Study in an orderly environment.
5. Put your notes on computer, so that they can readily be reorganized; print out each organization and compare them.

Linguistic Learners
Love words and new vocabulary.

Strategies to Take Advantage of Your "Linguistic" Style
1. When writing papers, come back to the paper and see what words you can get rid of (you probably have too many).
2. Take notes as you read, writing key points down; then study your notes, rather than the book, or you may have trouble focusing on key points.

Spatial Learners
Like fewer words and more boxes and diagrams.

Strategies to Take Advantage of Your "Spatial" Style
1. Put boxes around key information.
2. Diagram concepts you're trying to remember.
3. Recopy notes, using only key words.

Musical Learners
Like to hum, sing, play instruments.

Strategies to Take Advantage of Your "Musical" Style
1. Study while listening to favorite music. Remember what music you were listening to when studying specific content.
2. Go over information you want to remember in your head while playing an instrument.
3. Have someone read you the information while you're playing an instrument.

Appendix C
Recommended for Personal Application of Personality Type

For Hartman Personality Profile

Hartman, T. (1998). *The character code.* New York: Scribner.

Hartman, T. (1998). *The color code.* New York: Scribner.

Hartman, T. (1998). *The color code (audio tapes).* New York: Simon and Schuster Audio.

For Myers-Briggs Type Indicator

Hirsh, S., Kummerow, J. (1989). *Lifetypes.* New York: Warner Books.

Myers, I.B. (1987). *Introduction to type: A description of the theory and application of the Myers-Briggs type indicator.* Palo Alto, CA: Consulting Psychologists Press.

Myers, I.B., with Myers, P. (1995). *Gifts differing.* Palo Alto, CA: Consulting Psychologists Press.

Myers, I.B., with revisions by Myers, K., Kirby, L. (1993). *Introduction to type.* Palo Alto, CA: Consulting Psychologists Press.

Kroeger, O., Thuesen, J. (1988). *Type talk.* New York: Dell.

Quenk, N. (1993). *Beside ourselves: Our hidden personality in everyday life.* Palo Alto, CA: Consulting Psychologists Press.

For Pediatric and Youth Application

Hartman, T. (1990). *Hartman youth personality profile.* Midvale, UT: Color Code Communications.

Tieger, P., Barron-Tieger, B. (1997). *Nurture by nature: Understanding your child's personality type and becoming a better parent.* Boston: Little, Brown.

Examples of Critical Path, Data Base Assessment Tool, Neurological Focus Assessment Tool, Neurovascular Focus Assessment Tool

APPENDIX D—FRACTURED HIP CLINICAL PATHWAY

CARE NEED	DAY 4 - POD 2	Done	Var	DAY 5 - POD 3	Done	Var	DAY 6 - POD 4	Done	Var	DAY 7 - POD 5	Done	Var
ASSESSMENT	DATE: Neurovasc check q shift & prn *Sequential Compression Device *TED stockings-off 1 hr q shift Mentation clear; 02 prn; IS/CDB prn; breath sounds clear *02 sat. if new onset confusion < 90–notify MD ___ T < 38C; Skin check q shift *Change dressing ___ *DC wound drain			DATE: Neurovasc check q shift & prn *Sequential Compression Device *TED stockings-off 1 hr q shift Mentation clear Breath sounds clear T < 38 Dressing dry and intact/change prn Skin Intact			DATE: Neurovascular check q shift & prn *Sequential Compression Device *TED stockings-off 1 hr q shift Mentation clear Breath sounds clear T < 38 Dressing dry and intact/change prn Skin Intact			DATE: Neurovascular check q shift & prn *TED stockings-off 1 hr q shift Mentation clear T < 38C Dressing dry and intact/change prn Skin Intact		
PAIN	PO Meds Pharm consult if new confusion			PO Meds			PO Meds			PO Meds		
MOBILITY ENDO: NSG: PT:	Turn q 2-3 hrs while in bed with wedge Exercises per protocol Ambulate to chair OT consult, if necessary Weight Bearing Status:___ P.T.			Recliner × 1 (3-11) Wedge @ NOC Exercises per protocol Increase ambulation Start home exercise program ___ P.T.			Wedge prn/pillows Increase ambulation Exercises continued Increase ambulation Bathroom transfer ___ P.T.			Increase ambulation Exercises continued Increase ambulation Stairs/crutches, prn Car transfer @ D/C P.T.		
ORIF NSG: PT:	Transfer bed to chair w/2 assists Exercises per protocol Ambulate to chair O.T. referral, if necessary ___ P.T. ___ O.T.			Ambulate 3-11 Exercises per protocol Increase ambulation Bathroom transfer OT consult if necessary ___ O.T. Start home exercise program ___ P.T.			Increase ambulation Exercises continued Increase ambulation Stairs/crutches prn ADL Instruction prn ___ O.T. ___ P.T.			Increase ambulation Exercises continued Increase ambulation Stairs/crutches prn Discharge P.T.		
NUTRITION	DAT: took 50% HS Supplement ___ RN			DAT: took 75% HS Supplement ___ RN			DAT: took 75% HS Supplement ___ RN			Advance as tol.		
SELF-CARE	1/2 bath; assist w/HS care			Advance self care as tol.			Advance self care as tol.			Voiding qs		
ELIMINATION	*Foley; voiding qs; STOOL SOFTENER; laxative prn			*DC Foley/voiding qs; STOOL SOFTENER; Suppository if no BM 7-3			Voiding qs STOOL SOFTENER					
DISCHARGE PLANNING/ TEACHING	SWS evaluate discharge plan DC date Caregiver identified: Reinforce hip precautions prn Connections referral prn			Assess need for/order home equipment ORIF: Discharge Instructions ___ Mobility ___ Meds ___ ADL's Discuss role of nutrition in healing			DISCHARGE ORIF patient ENDO: Discharge Instructions ___ Mobility ___ Meds ___ ADL's			Discharge endoprosthesis patient		
LAB/ DIAGNOSTICS*	PTT if on prophylaxis**			PTT if on prophylaxis**						PTT if on prophylaxis**		

		D	E	N			D	E	N			D	E	N
	Init.	Signature			Init.	Signature			Init.	Signature			Init.	Signature	

Variance Codes
A-Not Indicated
B-Patient condition
C-Physician order override
D-Equipment/supplies
E-Pt/family decision
F-Family unavailable
G-Scheduling
H-Service not provided

I-Department closed
J-Placement availability
K-Docum. for DC
L-Physician DC plan
Z-Other

mac/xl/fhrpathway

© OHMC 5/24/93

*Physician order required

From Victor M. Goldberg, M.D., Department of Orthopedics, University Hospitals of Cleveland.

**THE BRYN MAWR HOSPITAL
NURSING DEPARTMENT**

NURSING ADMISSION ASSESSMENT

DATE _2/6/99_ TIME OF ARRIVAL _14:00_

FROM _ER_

ACCOMPANIED BY _friend_

VIA: WHEELCHAIR _____ STRETCHER _✓_ AMBULATORY _____

ID BRACELET _✓_ INFORMATION OBTAINED FROM _patient_

I. VITAL STATISTICS

TEMP _101_ PULSE _120_ RESP _30_

ORAL _✓_ RECTAL _____ AXILLARY _____

BP _^{1to}/90_ RA _143/86_ LA _138/88_ POSITION _sitting_

WEIGHT _148_ HEIGHT _5'6"_

SCALE: BED _____ CHAIR _____ STANDING _✓_

DEFERRED _____

ORIENTED TO ROOM _✓_

PROSTHESIS, APPLIANCES OR OTHER DEVICES: _0_

DENTURES _0_

FULL: UPPER _0_ LOWER _0_

PARTIAL: UPPER _0_ LOWER _0_

EYE GLASSES _✓_

CONTACT LENSES _✓_

HEARING AID _0_

OTHER _0_

COMMENTS _glasses and contacts in drawer_

PATIENT HAS BROUGHT TO HOSPITAL? YES _____ NO _____

EXCEPTIONS _____

*WALKER/CANE/CRUTCHES _____

*ARTIFICIAL LIMBS _____

*BRACES _____

*FALSE EYE _____

WIG _____

II. ALLERGIES: DRUGS _✓_ DYES _____ FOOD _✓_ OTHER _____ NONE KNOWN _____

SPECIFY AGENT	DESCRIBE REACTION (IF KNOWN)
Keflex	Rash
Tomatoes	Rash

III. HEALTH PERCEPTION-HEALTH MAINTENANCE

A. PRESENT ILLNESS:

1. ADMITTING DIAGNOSIS _Diabetes   R/o Kidney Infection_

2. REASON FOR ADMISSION (PATIENT'S STATEMENT) _"Fever for 4 days"_

3. DURATION OF PRESENT ILLNESS _4 days_

4. PAST AND PRESENT TREATMENT OF PRESENT ILLNESS AND RESPONSE _None_

5. PATIENT AWARE OF DIAGNOSIS: YES _✓_ NO _____ NOT ESTABLISHED _____

B. PREVIOUS ILLNESSES: (INCLUDING HOSPITALIZATION)

_Multiple admissions for diabetic control and
urinary tract infections_

C. ARE YOU TAKING ANY MEDICATIONS (PRESCRIBED OR OVER THE COUNTER) YES ✓ NO _____

MEDICATION	DOSE	WHEN DO YOU TAKE IT	WHY DO YOU TAKE IT	LAST DOSE	BROUGHT TO HOSPITAL YES	BROUGHT TO HOSPITAL NO	DISPOSITION
Tylenol	500mg	PRN	Fever / Aches	12:00		✓	—
Regular Insulin	5u	AC	Diabetes	8:00		✓	—

D. DO YOU OR HAVE YOU EVER USED?

	YES	NO	LAST USED	FREQUENCY/AMOUNT
ALCOHOL		✓		
RECREATIONAL DRUGS		✓		

E. DO YOU SMOKE? YES _____ PKS/DAY _____ HOW LONG _____

NO: DID YOU EVER SMOKE? NO ✓ YES ____ PKS/DAY _____ HOW LONG _____ WHEN DID YOU QUIT _____

IV. COGNITIVE PERCEPTUAL: HEADACHE yes SEIZURES 0 BLACKOUTS 0 DIZZINESS 0 NO C/O —

A. LEVEL OF CONSCIOUSNESS: ALERT ✓ DROWSY _____ RESPONDS TO: PAIN _____ VERBAL STIMULI _____ UNRESPONSIVE _____

B. ORIENTED: TIME ✓ PLACE ✓ PERSON ✓ COMMENTS —

C. MOOD: RELAXED _____ ANXIOUS ✓ SAD _____ ANGRY _____ WITHDRAWN _____ OTHER _____

D. RECENT MEMORY CHANGE: YES _____ NO ✓ SPECIFY _____

E. RESPONDS TO DIRECTIONS: YES ✓ NO _____ SPECIFY _____

F. SPEECH: CLEAR ✓ SLURRED _____ GARBLED _____ UNABLE TO SPEAK _____ APHASIC _____

G. LANGUAGE SPOKEN: ENGLISH ✓ OTHER _____

H. HEARING: WNL ✓ IMPAIRED _____ CORRECTED _____ DEAF _____ SIGN LANGUAGE _____ LIP READS _____

I. VISION: WNL ✓ IMPAIRED _____ CORRECTED ✓ BLIND _____

J. PAIN: YES ✓ NO _____ DESCRIBE headache, right flank pain

HOW DO YOU MANAGE YOUR PAIN? Tylenol

K. LEARNING READINESS: NO LIMITATIONS _____ WILLING TO LEARN ✓ RESISTS LEARNING _____

EMOTIONALLY READY TO LEARN: YES ✓ NO _____ REQUIRES CONCRETE LANGUAGE/REINFORCEMENT _____ FORGETFUL _____

TEACHING TO BE DIRECTED PRIMARILY TO patient

FAMILY MEMBER/SIGNIFICANT OTHER

L. COMMENTS Knowledgeable about diabetes

V. ROLE RELATIONSHIP (PSYCHOSOCIAL) / DISCHARGE PLANNING

A. OCCUPATION Teacher

B. LIVE ALONE ✓ WITH FAMILY _____ NURSING HOME _____ OTHER _____ COMMENT _____

C. DESCRIBE PHYSICAL ENVIRONMENT 2 story house

D. ANTICIPATED DISCHARGE TO: ECF _____ HOME CARE SERVICES _____

OTHER _____ HOME ✓ IF GOING HOME, WHO COULD HELP YOU WITH

HEALTHCARE NEEDS AFTER DISCHARGE? friends _____

E. DO YOU WISH TO SEE A MEMBER OF THE CLERGY WHILE YOU ARE HERE? YES _____ NO ✓ AFFILIATION _____

F. COMMENTS _____

VI. HEALTH HISTORY/ASSESSMENT

A. CARDIOVASCULAR: ANGINA 0 ARRHYTHMIA 0 MURMUR 0 EDEMA 0 PALPITATIONS 0

CHEST PAIN 0 MI 0 CVA 0 ANEURYSM 0 HYPERTENSION ✓

PACEMAKER 0 TYPE 0 NO C/O _____

PULSE: STRONG ✓ WEAK _____ REGULAR _____ IRREGULAR ✓

RIGHT DORSALIS PEDAL PULSE: STRONG ✓ WEAK _____ ABSENT _____

LEFT DORSALIS PEDAL PULSE: STRONG ✓ WEAK _____ ABSENT _____

COMMENTS _____

8183 PG 2 (REV 9/90)

B. RESPIRATORY: COUGH __0__ PRODUCTIVE __0__ PAIN __0__ DESCRIBE __0_____

FREQUENT COLDS __0__ HOARSENESS __0__ ASTHMA __0__ TB __0__ SOB: ON EXERTION __0__ AT REST __0__ NO C/O __✓__

COMMENTS _____

C. RENAL: KIDNEY STONES __✓__ INFECTIONS _____ RETENTION __✓__ BURNING __✓__ POLYURIA __✓__ DYSURIA _____ NO C/O _____

URINARY DEVICES? __0__ TYPE __0_____

INCONTINENCE __0__ DAYTME __0__ NOCTURNAL __0__ STRESS __0__

DO YOU GET UP DURING NIGHT TO URINATE? YES __✓__ NO _____

COMMENTS __Probable kidney infection_____

D. GASTROINTESTINAL (NUTRITION/METABOLIC)

1. HISTORY OF DIABETES? YES __✓__ NO _____ DO YOU TEST FOR SUGAR? YES __✓__ NO _____ URINE _____ BLOOD __✓__

DIET CONTROLLED _____ INSULIN DEPENDENT __✓__ ORAL HYPOGLYCEMICS _____

NUMBER OF YEARS __10__ PREVIOUS DIABETES EDUCATION: YES __✓__ NO _____

2. NUMBER OF MEALS/DAY __3__ SNACKS __2__ SPECIAL DIET __0_____

3. PATIENT'S ABILITY TO EAT: INDEPENDENT __✓__ WITH ASSISTANCE __0__ SPECIFY __0__

DIFFICULTY SWALLOWING __0__

4. WEIGHT CHANGE IN THE LAST SIX MONTHS: NONE __0__ LOST _____ LBS GAINED _____ LBS

5. DO YOU EXPERIENCE NAUSEA/VOMITING? YES __✓__ NO _____ RELATED TO __fever_____

6. DO YOU EXPERIENCE CRAMPING __0__ HEARTBURN __0__ RECTAL PAIN __0__ GAS __0__ LAST BM: __yesterday__

7. BOWEL: USUAL TIME: __10__ A.M. _____ P.M. FREQUENCY: DAILY _____ EVERY OTHER DAY __✓__ OTHER _____

INCONTINENCE __0__ DEVICES USED __0_____

COLOR: BROWN __✓__ CLAY-COLORED __0__ BLACK __0__ BLOOD __0__

CONSTIPATION: NONE _____ OCCASIONALLY __✓__ FREQUENTLY _____

DIARRHEA: NONE _____ OCCASIONALLY __✓__ FREQUENTLY _____ OSTOMY _____

LAXATIVES/ENEMAS USED/HOW OFTEN? (SPECIFY) __0_____

8. ABDOMEN: SOFT __✓__ NON-TENDER __✓__ NON-DISTENDED _____ FIRM _____ TENDER _____ DISTENDED _____

BOWEL SOUNDS: PRESENT __✓__ ABSENT _____

COMMENTS: _____

E. SKIN CONDITION

COLOR: WNL __✓__ PALE _____ CYANOTIC _____ JAUNDICE _____ OTHER _____

TEMP: WARM __✓__ COOL _____ TURGOR: WNL _____ POOR _____

EDEMA: NO __✓__ YES _____ DESCRIPTION/LOCATION _____

LESIONS: NO __✓__ YES _____ DESCRIPTION/LOCATION _____

DECUBITUS: NO __✓__ YES _____ LOCATION(S) _____ (SEE TISSUE TRAUMA FORM)

BRUISES: NO __✓__ YES _____ DESCRIPTION/LOCATION _____

RASHES: NO __✓__ YES _____ DESCRIPTION/LOCATION _____

REDNESS: NO __✓__ YES _____ DESCRIPTION/LOCATION _____

COMMENTS: _____

F. MUSCULO-SKELETAL: CRAMPING _____ ARTHRITIS _____ STIFFNESS __✓__ SWELLING _____ NO C/O _____

MOTOR FUNCTION: RIGHT ARM: WNL __✓__ AMPUTATED ___ SPASTIC ___ FLACCID ___ WEAKNESS ___ PARALYSIS ___ OTHER ___

LEFT ARM: WNL __✓__ AMPUTATED ___ SPASTIC ___ FLACCID ___ WEAKNESS ___ PARALYSIS ___ OTHER ___

RIGHT LEG: WNL __✓__ AMPUTATED ___ SPASTIC ___ FLACCID ___ WEAKNESS ___ PARALYSIS ___ OTHER ___

LEFT LEG: WNL __✓__ AMPUTATED ___ SPASTIC ___ FLACCID ___ WEAKNESS ___ PARALYSIS ___ OTHER ___

COMMENTS _Has some joint stiffness_ _____

VII. SLEEP-REST/ACTIVITY

A. USUAL SLEEP PATTERN: BEDTIME _____ HOURS SLEPT _____ NAPS: NO _____ ✓ YES _____

B. DIFFICULTY FALLING ASLEEP: NO __✓__ YES _____ SPECIFY _____

C. SLEEP AIDS USED: NO __✓__ YES _____ SPECIFY _____

D. DOES PATIENT HAVE DIFFICULTY/PROBLEMS IN:

BATHING: NO __✓__ YES _____ SPECIFY _____

DRESSING: NO __✓__ YES _____ SPECIFY _____

AMBULATING: NO __✓__ YES _____ BALANCE/GAIT: STEADY _____ UNSTEADY _____ TIRES EASILY _____ WEAKNESS _____

COMMENTS _independent_ _____

VIII. SEXUAL HEALTH (FEMALES)

A. LMP _2/1_ LAST PAP SMEAR _10/98_

B. DO YOU EXAMINE YOUR BREASTS? YES __✓__ NO _____ HOW OFTEN? _Every month_

C. IF NO, DO YOU KNOW HOW? YES _____ NO _____ WOULD YOU BE INTERESTED IN LEARNING? YES _____ NO _____

PAMPHLET GIVEN? YES _____ NO _____ COMMENTS _____

IX. ASSESSMENT SUMMARY: _Acutely ill female who manages home care well._

X. NURSING DIAGNOSES: _High Risk For Fluid Volume Deficit R/T fever and nausea._

XI. THE FOLLOWING SECTIONS WERE DEFERRED ON ADMISSION (IDENTIFY BY SECTION NUMBER): _None_

REASON: _____

DATE/TIME	COMPLETED BY	PRIMARY NURSE	DATE/TIME	REVIEWED BY PRIMARY NURSE
2/6/99 13:00	R Alfaro ___ RN	YES ✓ NO ___	___/___	_____ RN
___/___	_____ RN	YES ___ NO ___	___/___	_____ RN

8183 PG 4 (REV 9/90)

THE BRYN MAWR HOSPITAL
NURSING DEPARTMENT

NEUROLOGICAL ASSESSMENT SHEET

1MM	2MM	3MM	4MM	5MM	6MM	7MM	8MM	9MM
•	•	•	•	●	●	●	●	●

	DATE		2/12/99	2/12	2/12	2/12										
	TIME			1:00	9:00	17:00										
V I T A L S	**BLOOD PRESSURE**			120/70	110/70	113/68									**RESPIRATORY TYPE**	
	PULSE			74	80	72									N = NORMAL	
	TEMPERATURE			98	98	98									CS = CHEYNE STOKES	
	RESPIRATORY RATE			20	22	20									SH = SUSTAINED HYPERVENTILATION	
	RESPIRATORY TYPE			N	N	N										
C O M A S C A L E	**EYES OPEN**	SPONTANEOUSLY 4													E = EYES CLOSED BY SWELLING	
		TO COMMAND 3		✓	✓	✓										
		TO PAIN 2														
		NO RESPONSE 1														
	BEST MOTOR RESPONSE	OBEYS COMMANDS 6		✓	✓	✓									RECORD BEST ARM RESPONSE	
		LOCALIZES PAIN 5														
		FLEXION WITHDRAWAL 4														
		FLEXION (ABNORMAL) 3														
		EXTENSION (ABNORMAL) 2														
		NO RESPONSE 1														
	BEST VERBAL RESPONSE	ORIENTED 5			✓	✓									T = ENDOTRACHEAL TUBE OR TRACHEOSTOMY	
		CONFUSED 4		✓												
		INAPPROPRIATE WORDS 3														
		INCOMPREHENSIBLE SOUNDS 2														
		NO RESPONSE 1													A = APHASIA	
	TOTAL SCORE			13	14	14										
P U P I L S	**SIZE**	R		7	6	7									B = BRISK S = SLUGGISH	
	REACTION			5	B	B									N = NO REACTION C = CLOSED	
	SIZE	L		7	6	7									SC = SUSTAINED CONSTRICTION 2°	
	REACTION			B	B	B									CATARACT SURGERY	
L I M B M O V E M E N T	**GRADE LIMB SPONTANEOUS OR TO COMMAND. DO NOT RATE REFLEX MOVEMENT**	RA		5	5	5									LIMB MOVEMENT SCALE 0 = PARALYSIS	
		RL		5	5	5									1 = VISIBLE MUSCLE CONTRACTION; NO MOVEMENT	
		LA		5	5	5									2 = WEAK CONTRACTION; NOT ENOUGH TO OVERCOME GRAVITY	
		LL		5	5	5										
L I M B S E N S A T I O N	**DULL**	RA		N	N	N									3 = MOVE AGAINST GRAVITY; NOT EXTERNAL RESISTANCE	
		RL		N	N	N									4 = NORMAL ROM; CAN BE OVERCOME BY INCREASED GRAVITY	
		LA		N	N	N										
		LL		N	N	N									5 = NORMAL MUSCLE STRENGTH	
	SHARP	RA		N	N	N									SENSATION CODES N = NORMAL	
		RL		N	N	N									D = DECREASED	
		LA		N	N	N									A = ABSENT	
		LL		N	N	N										
	SEIZURE ACTIVITY			A	A	A									A = ABSENT P = PRESENT	
	GAG REFLEX			P	P	P									A = ABSENT P = PRESENT	
	INITIALS															

SIGNATURE	INITIALS	SIGNATURE	INITIALS
R. Alfaro RN	RA		
C. Sebhrist RN	CS		
a. Carlson	AC		

F8064
(REV 1/91)

THE BRYN MAWR HOSPITAL
NURSING SERVICE

NEURO-VASCULAR ASSESSMENT FLOW SHEET

EXTREMITY(IES) TO BE ASSESSED: Left lower leg

FREQUENCY OF ASSESSMENT: q8h

TYPE OF EXTERNAL SUPPORT: Cast

Date	Time	Hospital Day / Post-Op Day	Limb	Color	Capillary Refill	Temp.	Edema	Sensation	Numbness & Tingling	Motion	Pulse	Proprioception	Comments	Signature
2/1/99	9:00	1 / 0	LE	Pink	R	W	P	P	N	P	P	P	Toes slightly edematous	R. Alfaro RN
2/1/99	17:00	1 / 0	✓	✓	✓	✓	A	P	A	✓	✓	✓	Moves toes well	C. Sechrist RN
2/2/99	1:00	2 / 1	✓	✓	✓	✓	✓	✓	✓	✓	✓	✓	Med for incisional pain	a. Carlson RN

KEY

Limb(s): Specify RUE, LUE, RLE, LLE
Color: Pink, Pale, Cyanotic
Capillary Refill: Rapid, Slow
Temperature: Warm, Cool, Cold
Edema: Absent (A), Present(P)
Sensation: Absent (A), Decreased (D), Present (P)

Numbness (N), Tingling (T): Present (P),
    Decreased (D), Absent (A)
Motion: Present (P), Decreased (D), Absent (A)
Pulses: Present (P), Absent (A)
Proprioception: Present (P), Absent (A)
NA: Not Applicable
*: See Nurses Notes

FORM 8066

Health Perception–Health Management Pattern

Adult Failure to Thrive
Altered Development, Risk for
Aspiration, Risk for
Autonomic Dysreflexia, Risk for
Delayed Surgical Recovery
Growth and Development, Altered
Growth, Risk for Altered
Health Maintenance, Altered
Health-Seeking Behaviors
Injury, Risk for
Management of Therapeutic Regimen (Individual), Ineffective
Noncompliance
Poisoning, Risk for
Suffocation, Risk for
Trauma, Risk for

Nutritional-Metabolic Pattern

Body Temperature, Risk for Altered
   Hypothermia
   Hyperthermia
   Thermoregulation, Ineffective
Dentition, Altered
Fluid Volume Deficit
Fluid Volume Excess
Fluid Volume Imbalance, Risk for

From North American Nursing Diagnosis Association. (1999). NANDA nursing diagnoses: Definitions and classifications 1992–2000. Philadelphia: Author.

Infection, Risk for
Latex Allergy
Latex Allergy, Risk for
Nausea
Nutrition, Altered: Less than Body Requirements
   Breastfeeding, Effective
   Breastfeeding, Ineffective
   Breastfeeding, Interrupted
   Feeding Pattern, Ineffective Infant
Nutrition, Altered: More than Body Requirements
Nutrition, Altered: Risk for More than Body Requirements
Oral Mucous Membrane, Altered
Protection, Altered
Skin Integrity, Impaired
Swallowing, Impaired
Tissue Integrity, Impaired

Elimination Pattern

Bowel Incontinence
Constipation
   Perceived Constipation
Constipation, Risk for
Diarrhea
Urinary Elimination, Altered Patterns of
   Incontinence, Functional
   Incontinence, Stress
   Incontinence, Total
   Incontinence, Urge
   Urinary Retention
Urinary Urge Incontinence, Risk for

Activity-Exercise Pattern
Activity Intolerance
Activity Intolerance, Risk for
Airway Clearance, Ineffective
Bed Mobility, Impaired
Breathing Pattern, Ineffective
Cardiac Output, Decreased
Disorganized Infant Behavior
Disuse Syndrome
Diversional Activity Deficit
Gas Exchange, Impaired
Fatigue
Home Maintenance Management, Impaired
Mobility, Impaired Physical
Peripheral Neurovascular Dysfunction, Risk for
Self-Care Deficit, Bathing/Hygiene
Self-Care Deficit, Dressing/Grooming
Self-Care Deficit, Feeding
Self-Care Deficit, Toileting
Tissue Perfusion, Altered (Specify) renal, cerebral, cardiopulmonary, gastrointestinal, peripheral
Ventilation, Inability to Sustain Spontaneous
Ventilatory Weaning Response, Dysfunctional
Walking, Impaired
Wheelchair Mobility, Impaired
Wheelchair Transfer Ability, Impaired

Sleep-Rest Pattern
Sleep Deprivation
Sleep Pattern Disturbance

Cognitive-Perceptual Pattern
Conflict, Decisional (Specify)
Knowledge Deficit (Specify)
Pain
Pain, Chronic
Sensory/Perceptual Alterations (Specify) visual, auditory, kinesthetic, gustatory, tactile, olfactory)

Thought Process, Altered
Unilateral Neglect

Self-Perception/Self-Concept Pattern
Anxiety
Body Image Disturbance
Chronic Sorrow
Death Anxiety
Fear
Hopelessness
Personal Identity Disturbance
Powerlessness
Self-Esteem Disturbance
Self-Esteem Disturbance, Chronic, Low
Self-Esteem Disturbance, Situational Low

Role-Relationship Pattern
Communication, Impaired*
Communication, Impaired Verbal
Family Processes, Altered
Grieving*
Grieving, Anticipatory
Grieving, Dysfunctional
Parenting, Altered
Parenting, Risk for Altered
Parental Role Conflict
Role Performance, Altered
Social Interaction, Impaired
Social Isolation

Sexual-Reproductive Pattern
Sexual Dysfunction
Sexuality Patterns, Altered

Coping–Stress Tolerance Pattern
Adjustment, Impaired
Caregiver Role Strain

---

*These diagnoses are not on the NANDA list as of 1999 but have been added by the author.

Coping, Ineffective Individual
  Defensive Coping
  Ineffective Denial
Coping: Compromised, Ineffective Family
Coping: Disabling, Ineffective Family
Coping: Potential for Growth, Family
Post-Trauma Syndrome
Post-Trauma Syndrome, Risk for

Rape Trauma Syndrome
Relocation Stress Syndrome
Self-Mutilation, Risk for
Violence, Risk for

Value-Belief Pattern
Spiritual Distress
Spiritual Distress, Risk for

Appendix F

American Nurses Association Standards for Practice, American Nurses Association Code for Nurses, and a Patient's Bill of Rights

AMERICAN NURSES ASSOCIATION STANDARDS FOR PRACTICE

Standards of Care (Use of the Nursing Process)

Standard I   Assessment: The nurse collects client health data.

II   Diagnosis: The nurse analyzes assessment data in determining diagnoses.

III   Outcome Identification: The nurse identifies expected outcomes individualized to the client.

IV   Planning: The nurse develops a plan of care that prescribes interventions to attain expected outcomes.

V   Implementation: The nurse implements the interventions identified in the plan of care.

VI   Evaluation: The nurse evaluates the client's progress toward attainment of outcomes.

Standards of Professional Performance (Professional Behavior)

Standard I   Quality of Care: The nurse systematically evaluates the quality and effectiveness of nursing practice.

II   Performance Appraisal: The nurse evaluates his/her own nursing practice in relation to professional practice standards and relevant statutes and regulations.

III   Education: The nurse acquires and maintains current knowledge in nursing practice.

IV   Collegiality: The nurse contributes to the professional development of peers, colleagues, and others.

V   Ethics: The nurse's decisions and actions on behalf of clients are determined in an ethical manner.

VI   Collaboration: The nurse collaborates with the client, significant others, and health-care providers in providing client care.

VII   Research: The nurse uses research findings in practice.

VIII   Resource Utilization: The nurse considers factors related to safety, effectiveness, and cost in planning and delivering client care.

Reprinted with permission from *Standards of Clinical Nursing Practice.* © 1991, American Nurses Association, Washington, DC.

AMERICAN NURSES ASSOCIATION CODE FOR NURSES

1. The nurse provides services with respect for human dignity and the uniqueness of the client unrestricted by considerations of social or economic status, personal attributes, or the nature of health problems.
2. The nurse safeguards the client's right to privacy by judiciously protecting information of a confidential nature.
3. The nurse acts to safeguard the client and the public when health care and safety are affected by the incompetent, unethical, or illegal practice of any person.
4. The nurse assumes responsibility and accountability for individual nursing judgments and actions.
5. The nurse maintains competence in nursing.
6. The nurse exercises informed judgment and uses individual competence and qualifications as criteria in seeking consultation, accepting responsibilities, and delegating nursing activities to others.
7. The nurse participates in activities that contribute to the ongoing development of the profession's body of knowledge.
8. The nurse participates in the profession's efforts to implement and improve standards of nursing.
9. The nurse participates in the profession's efforts to establish and maintain conditions of employment conducive to high quality nursing care.
10. The nurse participates in the profession's effort to protect the public from misinforma-

tion and misrepresentation and to maintain the integrity of nursing.
11. The nurse collaborates with members of the health professions and other citizens in promoting community and national efforts to meet the health needs of the public.

A PATIENT'S BILL OF RIGHTS

Introduction

Effective health care requires collaboration between patients and physicians and other health care professionals. Open and honest communication, respect for personal and professional values, and sensitivity to differences are integral to optimal patient care. As the setting for the provision of health services, hospitals must provide a foundation for understanding and respecting the rights and responsibilities of patients, their families, physicians, and other caregivers. Hospitals must ensure a health care ethic that respects the role of patients in decision making about treatment choices and other aspects of their care. Hospitals must be sensitive to cultural, racial, linguistic, religious, age, gender, and other differences as well as the needs of persons with disabilities.

The American Hospital Association presents *A Patient's Bill of Rights* with the expectation that it will contribute to more effective patient care and be supported by the hospital on behalf of the institution, its medical staff, employees, and patients. The American Hospital Association encourages health care institutions to tailor this bill of rights to their patient community by translat-

---

Reprinted with permission from *Code for Nurses with Interpretive Statements,* © 1985, American Nurses Association, Washington, DC.

A Patient's Bill of Rights was first adopted by the American Hospital Association in 1973. This revision was approved by the AHA Board of Trustees on October 21, 1992.

Reprinted with permission of the American Hospital Association, copyright 1992.

ing and/or simplifying the language of this bill of rights as may be necessary to ensure that patients and their families understand their rights and responsibilities.

Bill of Rights*

1. The patient has the right to considerate and respectful care.
2. The patient has the right to and is encouraged to obtain from physicians and other direct caregivers relevant, current, and understandable information concerning diagnosis, treatment, and prognosis.

    Except in emergencies when the patient lacks decision-making capacity and the need for treatment is urgent, the patient is entitled to the opportunity to discuss and request information related to the specific procedures and/or treatments, the risks involved, the possible length of recuperation, and the medically reasonable alternatives and their accompanying risks and benefits.

    Patients have the right to know the identity of physicians, nurses, and others involved in their care, as well as when those involved are students, residents, or other trainees. The patient also has the right to know the immediate and long-term financial implications of treatment choices, insofar as they are known.
3. The patient has the right to make decisions about the plan of care prior to and during the course of treatment and to refuse a recommended treatment or plan of care to the extent permitted by law and hospital policy and to be informed of the medical consequences

of this action. In case of such refusal, the patient is entitled to other appropriate care and services that the hospital provides or transfer to another hospital. The hospital should notify patients of any policy that might affect patient choice within the institution.

4. The patient has the right to have an advance directive (such as a living will, health care proxy, or durable power of attorney for health care) concerning treatment or designating a surrogate decision maker with the expectation that the hospital will honor the intent of that directive to the extent permitted by law and hospital policy.

    Health care institutions must advise patients of their rights under state law and hospital policy to make informed medical choices. They must ask if the patient has an advance directive, and include that information in patient records. The patient has the right to timely information about hospital policy that may limit its ability to implement fully a legally valid advance directive.
5. The patient has the right to every consideration of privacy. Case discussion, consultation, examination, and treatment should be conducted so as to protect each patient's privacy.
6. The patient has the right to expect that all communications and records pertaining to his/her care will be treated as confidential by the hospital, except in cases such as suspected abuse and public health hazards when reporting is permitted or required by law. The patient has the right to expect that the hospital will emphasize the confidentiality of this information when it releases it to any other parties entitled to review information in these records.
7. The patient has the right to review the records pertaining to his/her medical care and to have the information explained or in-

---

*These rights can be exercised on the patient's behalf by a designated surrogate or proxy decision maker if the patient lacks decision-making capacity, is legally incompetent, or is a minor.

terpreted as necessary, except when restricted by law.

8. The patient has the right to expect that, within its capacity and policies, a hospital will make reasonable response to the request of a patient for appropriate and medically indicated care and services. The hospital must provide evaluation, service, and/or referral as indicated by the urgency of the case. When medically appropriate and legally permissible, or when a patient has so requested, a patient may be transferred to another facility. The institution to which the patient is to be transferred must first have accepted the patient for transfer. The patient must also have the benefit of complete information and explanation concerning the need for, risks, benefits, and alternatives to such a transfer.

9. The patient has the right to ask and be informed of the existence of business relationships among the hospital, educational institutions, other health care providers, or payers that may influence the patient's treatment and care.

10. The patient has the right to consent to or decline to participate in proposed research studies or human experimentation affecting care and treatment or requiring direct patient involvement, and to have those studies fully explained prior to consent. A patient who declines to participate in research or experimentation is entitled to the most effective care that the hospital can otherwise provide.

11. The patient has the right to expect reasonable continuity of care when appropriate and to be informed by physicians and other caregivers of available and realistic patient care options when hospital care is no longer appropriate.

12. The patient has the right to be informed of hospital policies and practices that relate to patient care, treatment, and responsibilities. The patient has the right to be informed of available resources for resolving disputes, grievances, and conflicts, such as ethics committees, patient representatives, or other mechanisms available in the institution. The patient has the right to be informed of the hospital's charges for services and available payment methods.

The collaborative nature of health care requires that patients, or their families/surrogates, participate in their care. The effectiveness of care and patient satisfaction with the course of treatment depend, in part, on the patient's fulfilling certain responsibilities. Patients are responsible for providing information about past illnesses, hospitalizations, medications, and other matters related to health status. To participate effectively in decision making, patients must be encouraged to take responsibility for requesting additional information or clarification about their health status or treatment when they do not fully understand information and instructions. Patients are also responsible for ensuring that the health care institution has a copy of their written advance directive if they have one. Patients are responsible for informing their physicians and other caregivers if they anticipate problems in following prescribed treatment.

Patients should also be aware of the hospital's obligation to be reasonably efficient and equitable in providing care to other patients and the community. The hospital's rules and regulations are designed to help the hospital meet this obligation. Patients and their families are responsible for making reasonable accommodations to the needs of the hospital, other patients, medical staff, and hospital employees. Patients are responsible for providing necessary information for insurance claims and for working with the hospital to make payment arrangements, when necessary.

A person's health depends on much more than health care services. Patients are responsible for recognizing the impact of their lifestyle on their personal health.

Conclusion

Hospitals have many functions to perform, including the enhancement of health status, health promotion, and the prevention and treatment of injury and disease; the immediate and ongoing care and rehabilitation of patients; the education of health professionals, patients, and the community; and research. All these activities must be conducted with an overriding concern for the values and dignity of patients.

Mind Mapping: Getting in the "Right" State of Mind

WHAT IS MIND MAPPING?

Mind mapping is a method of documenting that uses the *right* brain (creative hemisphere) to enhance your ability to understand information and solve problems. Unlike outlining, which uses the *left* brain (logical hemisphere), mind mapping is flexible, has few rules, and is easy to learn and teach. The boxes on the next page compare right and left brain function and give steps for how to mind map; page 273 shows an example mind map.

WHEN DO YOU USE IT?

You can use it for a variety of purposes. Following are some of the most common:

- Taking notes/learning new content
- Writing papers/preparing presentations
- Preparing for exams
- Promoting idea generation (brainstorming)
- Facilitating group problem solving

WHAT ARE THE BENEFITS?

General benefits and specific group benefits follow:

General Benefits
- **Quicker** than regular note taking
- **Highlights** key ideas/gets rid of the irrelevant
- **Helps** you quickly gather, review, and recall large amounts of information
- **Increases** brain power available for *learning and problem solving* by reducing energy used on concerns about structure and documentation
- **Encourages** you to identify relationships and use creativity

Group Benefits
- **Promotes** communication (keeps everyone focused on the main issues)
- **Facilitates** problem solving (generates more ideas, helps group suspend judgment)
- **Makes** ideas and relationships clear

HOW DOES IT PROMOTE CRITICAL THINKING?

By pushing you to use your *right* brain talents, mind mapping facilitates the "productive phase" of critical thinking—the phase when you need to gather relevant information, identify relationships, and *produce* new ideas. Once you've completed this productive phase, you can get in touch with your *left* brain talents and move to the "judgment phase"—you can evaluate what your mind has *produced*, make *judgments* about its accuracy and usefulness, and make refinements.

Left Versus Right Hemisphere Function

Left Brain (Logical, Judging, Evaluating)	Right Brain (Creative, Idea Generating)
Deals with:	*Deals with:*
Language	Images/imagination
Logic	Colors/geometry
Linearity (step-by-step approaches)	Pattern, face, and map recognition
Numbers and sequence	Rhythm/music
Analysis	Dimension
	Parallel processing

Eight Steps for Mind Mapping to Promote Critical Thinking

1. **Put central theme or concept** in the center, bottom, or top of the page and draw a circle around it (see an example mind map below).
2. **Place the main ideas relating to the concept** on lines (or in circles) around the central theme.
3. **Add details** by putting them on lines (or in circles) connecting them to the main ideas.

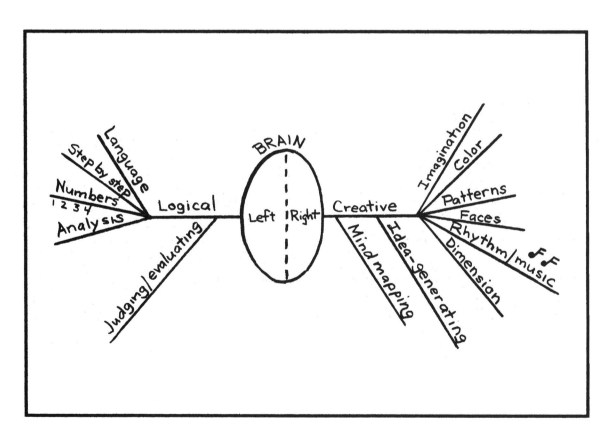

Mind Map of How the Brain Works
Adapted from Menthey, M., Miller, D. (1991). Tools for leaders, tools for managers. *Nursing Management, 22,* 2–21, with permission of Springhouse Corporation.®

4. **Use key words or simple pictures** only; keep it legible.
5. **Make sure no idea stands alone.** If you can't connect an idea with something on the page, it's irrelevant to the central theme.
6. **Don't allow yourself to slow down** over concerns about where to place words (this is your left brain habits trying to dominate). Rather, let your ideas flow and use lines to show connections.
7. **Use colors** to highlight the most important ideas.
8. **Once you've completed your mind map,** get in touch with your left brain talents (judging and evaluating) and evaluate what you've produced. **Revise as needed.**

Glossary

advanced practice nurse A nurse who, by virtue of credentials (usually completion of a masters program and certification), has a wide scope of authority to act (may include treating medical problems and prescribing medications).

air embolism An air bubble that gets into the bloodstream. Can be fatal.

analysis A mental process in which one seeks to get a better understanding of the nature of something by carefully separating the whole into smaller parts. For example, if you want to know more about someone's physical health, you examine each organ and system separately.

anaphylactic shock Extreme hypotension caused by an allergic reaction; requires immediate treatment or can be fatal.

assessment tool A printed or computerized form used to ensure that key information is gathered and recorded during assessment.

assumption Something that's taken for granted without proof. (Compare with *hypothesis* and *inference.*)

attitude A way of acting, feeling, or thinking that shows one's disposition, opinion, etc. (e.g., a threatening attitude).

baseline data Information that describes the status of a problem before treatment begins.

benchmark A standard or point in measuring quality. In health care, benchmarks are determined by analyzing the data collected over a period of time.

best practices A term referring to ways certain problems are best prevented and managed from an outcome and cost perspective.

care variance When a patient hasn't achieved activities or outcomes by the time frame noted on a critical path.

caring behavior Behavior that shows understanding and respect for another's perceptions, feelings, needs, and desires.

circumstances The conditions or facts attending an event or having some bearing on it.

classify To arrange or group together data according to categories, thereby increasing understanding because relationships become more obvious.

client-centered outcome (1) A statement that describes the benefits the client is expected to experience from nursing care. (2) A statement or phrase that describes what the client or patient is expected to be able to do when the plan of care is terminated. For example, Will be discharged home able to walk independently using a walker by 8/24.

clinical judgment (1) Nursing opinion(s) made about a person's, family's, or group's health at a certain point in time. (2) Nursing decisions made about things like what to assess, what health data suggest, what to do first, and who should do it.

clinical reasoning See *clinical judgment.*

collaborative actions Nursing actions prescribed by a physician or facility protocol. For example, administering IVs. (Compare with *independent nursing actions.*)

competence The quality of having the necessary knowledge, skill, and attitude to perform an action.

context The circumstances in which a particular event occurs.

critical Characterized by careful and exact evaluation; crucial.

cues See *data.*

data Pieces of information about health status (e.g., vital signs).

data base assessment Comprehensive data collected when the client first enters the health care facility to gain information about all aspects of the health status.

data base form See *assessment tool.*

deductive reasoning Drawing *specific* conclusions from general principles and rules. For example, Since it's true that bacteria are killed by antibiotics, Jane's bacterial infection requires treatment with antibiotics. (Compare with *inductive reasoning.*)

defining characteristics The signs and symptoms usually associated with a specific nursing diagnosis.

definitive diagnosis The most specific, most correct diagnosis.

definitive interventions The most specific actions required to prevent, resolve, or control a health problem.

diagnose To make a judgment and identify and name actual problems or strengths after careful analysis of evidence from an assessment.

diagnostic error When a health problem has been overlooked or incorrectly identified.

diagnostic reasoning A method of thinking that involves specific, deliberate use of critical thinking to reach conclusions about health status.

diagnostic statement A phrase that clearly describes a diagnosis; includes the problem name, related (risk) factors, and any evidence confirming the diagnosis.

diaphoretic The condition of being sweaty, usually suspected to be a sign of a health problem (e.g., shock, disease).

disposition One's customary frame of mind or manner of response.

diuretic A drug given to enhance kidney function, thereby increasing fluid elimination from the body.

efficiency The quality of being able to produce a desired effect safely, with minimal risks, expense, and unnecessary effort.

emboli More than one embolus. (See *embolus.*)

embolus A clot that has moved through one vessel and lodged in another, reducing or totally blocking blood supply to tissues usually nourished by the vessels involved. (Compare with *thrombus.*)

empathy Understanding another's feelings or perceptions but not sharing the same feelings or point of view. (Compare with *sympathy.*)

empiric Relying solely on practical experience, ignoring science.

epidemiology The body of knowledge reflecting what is known about a specific health state.

esthetics A sense of what is pleasing to the eye.

ethics The study of the general nature of morals and of the specific moral choices to be made by individuals in relationships with others.

etiology The cause or contributing factors of a health problem.

expected outcome See client-centered outcome.

expedite To make something happen in a quick fashion.

explicit Clearly and specifically expressed or described.

focus assessment Data collection that aims to

gain specific information about only one aspect of health status.

guidelines Documents that delineate how care is to be provided in specific situations.

habits of inquiry Habits that enhance the ability to search for the truth (e.g., following rules of logic).

human responses Reactions of individuals or groups to health care concerns. For example, a woman may react to being told she is diabetic by feeling overwhelmed and unable to cope, or she may react by wanting to learn more about diabetes.

humanistic A way of thought or action concerned with the interests or ideals of people.

hypothesis (1) A hunch. (2) An assertion subject to verification or proof. (Compare with *assumption* and *inference.*)

imply To suggest by logical necessity.

independent nursing actions Nursing actions performed independently, without need for physician's orders or facility protocols. For example, ensuring adequate oral intake to prevent dehydration. (Compare with *collaborative actions.*)

independent nursing intervention See independent nursing actions.

indicator A criterion for evaluating progress toward a goal.

infer To suspect something or to attach meaning to information. For example, if someone is frowning, we may infer that he or she is worried.

inference Something we suspect to be true, based on a logical conclusion after examination of the evidence. (Compare with *assumption* and *hypothesis.*)

intervention Something done to prevent, cure, or control a health problem (e.g., turning someone every 2 hours is an intervention to prevent skin breakdown).

intubation The process of inserting a tube into an individual's bronchus to facilitate breathing.

intuition Knowing something without evidence.

irrigate To flush a tube (with normal saline solution or water) to keep it patent.

life processes Events or changes that occur during one's lifetime (e.g., growing up, getting married, losing someone).

logic A system of reasoning that leads to valid conclusions.

malpractice The negligent conduct of a person acting within his professional capacity.

measurable Capable of being clearly observed so that the quality or quantity of something can be determined.

medical domain Actions a physician is legally qualified to perform.

mentor A knowledgeable, insightful, and trusted person who helps someone else clarify thinking.

moral Concerned with the judgment of whether a human action or character is right or wrong.

myocardial infarction Partial or complete occlusion of one or more of the coronary arteries, causing death of coronary tissue.

nasogastric tube A tube inserted through the nose, down the esophagus, and into the stomach.

negligence Failure to provide the degree of care that someone of ordinary prudence would provide under the same circumstances. To claim negligence, it is necessary that there be a duty owed by one person to another, that the duty be breached, and that the breach cause harm.

nursing actions Behaviors of nurses in practice.

nursing intervention Action taken by a nurse to produce a nursing outcome.

nursing domain Actions a nurse is legally qualified to perform.

objective data Information that you can clearly observe or measure. For example, a pulse of 140 beats per minute.

outcome The expected result of interventions.

outcome measure A change, or absence of change, in a diagnosis.

paradigm (pa'-ra-dim) A model or way of doing things.

patent Open, so as to allow the flow of fluid or air.

phenomena Factors influencing humans that are concerns of nursing at a point further along in time dimension.

policies See *guidelines.*

potential diagnosis A problem or diagnosis that may occur because of certain risk factors present (e.g., someone who's on prolonged bed rest has a potential [or risk] for Impaired Skin Integrity).

potential problem See *potential diagnosis.*

preceptor An experienced, more qualified nurse assigned by a facility to facilitate learning for a less experienced nurse.

proactive (comes from *act before*) A way of thinking and behaving that accepts responsibility for one's actions and takes initiative to plan ahead to anticipate and prevent problems before they happen.

procedures See *guidelines.*

protocols See *guidelines.*

pulmonary embolus A clot that has blocked off circulation and oxygenation to lung tissue. Considered to be life-threatening.

QA See *quality assessment.*

QI See *quality improvement.*

qualified Having the competence and authority to perform an action.

quality The degree to which patient care services increase the probability of achieving *desired* outcomes with the decreased probability of *undesired* outcomes.

quality assessment (QA) Ongoing studies designed to evaluate quality of patient care and services. Just as assessment is the first step of the nursing process, QA is the first step of QI (quality improvement).

quality care Health care services that increase the probability of achieving *desired* results with decreased probability of *undesired* results.

quality improvement (QI) Ongoing studies designed to identify ways to promote achievement of desired outcomes in a timely, cost-effective fashion while decreasing the risks for undesired outcomes.

rales Abnormal breath sounds (crackles) caused by the passage of air through bronchi containing fluid. This sign is frequently associated with congestive heart failure.

related factor See *risk factor.*

response A reaction of an organism or person to a specific mechanism.

risk factor Something known to contribute to (or be associated with) a specific problem. (See also *etiology.*)

risk nursing diagnosis Human response to health conditions or life processes that may develop in a vulnerable individual, family, or community. Supported by risk factors that contribute to increased vulnerability (NANDA, 1997).*

signs Objective data that cause you to suspect a health problem.

somnolent Overly sleepy; difficult to arouse.

standards of care See *guidelines.*

---

*North American Nursing Diagnosis Association. (1997). *NANDA nursing diagnoses: Definitions and classifications 1997–1998.* Philadelphia: Author.

standard of nursing care The degree of skill, care, and diligence exercised by members of the nursing profession practicing in the same or a similar locality. Many states refer to standards in their nurse practice acts.

subjective data Information the patient states or communicates; the patient's perceptions. For example, My heart feels like it's racing.

sympathy Sharing the same feelings as another. (Compare with *empathy.*)

symptoms Subjective data that cause you to suspect a health problem.

synthesis The process of putting pieces of information together to make a whole. For example, nurses put individual signs and symptoms together to make a diagnosis.

thrombi More than one thrombus. (See *thrombus.*)

thrombus A clot that threatens blood supply to tissues. If the clot moves, it becomes an *embolus.*

tubal ligation Surgery performed to sterilize a woman by cutting and suturing her fallopian tubes.

validation The process of gathering more data to determine whether the information or data you've already collected are factual or true.

validity The extent to which something can be believed to be factual and true.

variance in care See *care variance.*

wellness diagnosis A clinical judgment about an individual, family, or community in transition from a specific level of wellness to a higher level of wellness (NANDA, 1997).*

*North American Nursing Diagnosis Association. (1997). *NANDA nursing diagnoses: Definitions and classifications 1997–1998.* Philadelphia: Author.

Comprehensive Bibliography

NOTE: Citations are presented alphabetically according to the following categories: Critical thinking in nursing • culture and diversity • general critical thinking • moral and ethical reasoning • nursing research and quality improvement • teaching, learning, and test taking.

Critical Thinking in Nursing

Abruzzese, R. (1996). *Nursing staff develoment* (2nd ed.). St. Louis, MO: Mosby–Year Book.

Adams, M., Whitlow, J., Stover, L., Johnson, K. (1996). Critical thinking as an educational outcome: An evaluation of current tools of measurement. *Nurse Educator, 21*(3), 23–31, 110–118.

Alfaro-LeFevre, R. (1998). *Applying nursing process* (4th ed.). Philadelphia, PA: Lippincott-Raven.

Alfaro-LeFevre, R. (1998). Improving your ability to think critically. *Nursing Spectrum (Greater Philadelphia/Tri-State Ed.), 7*(4), 12–14.

American Nurses Association. (1995). *A social policy statement.* Washington, DC: Author.

American Nurses Association. (1991). *Standards of clinical nursing practice.* Washington, DC: Author.

Anderson, S., Koch, M., Basset, S. (1998). *Health care resource management: Present and future challenges.* St. Louis, MO: Mosby.

Arnold, E., Boggs, K. (1994). *Interpersonal relationships: Professional communication skills for nurses* (2nd ed.). Philadelphia, PA: W.B. Saunders.

Bandman, E., Bandman, B. (1995). *Critical thinking in nursing* (2nd ed.). Norwalk, CT: Appleton & Lange.

Beck, S., Bennett, A., McLeod, R., Molyneaux, L. (1992). Review of research on critical thinking. in nursing education. In L. Allen (Ed.), *Review of re-search in nursing education* (vol. 5). New York, NY: National League for Nursing.

Becker, H. (1994). Indicators of critical thinking, communication, and therapeutic interventions among first line nursing supervisors. *Nurse Educator, 19*(2), 15–19.

Benner, P. (1984). *From novice to expert.* Menlo Park, CA: Addison-Wesley.

Black, J.M., Matassarin-Jacobs, E. (1997). *Medical-surgical nursing* (5th ed.). Philadelphia, PA: W.B. Saunders.

Boivin, J. (1997). There's no room for error. *Nursing Spectrum (FL Ed.), 7*(7), 3, 17.

Boucher, M. (1998). Delegation alert! *American Journal of Nursing, 98*(2), 26–32.

Bowers, B. (1993). Developing analytic thinking skills in early undergraduate education. *Journal of Nursing Education, 32*(3), 107–114.

Brigham, C. (1993). Nursing education and critical thinking: Interplay of content and thinking. *Holistic Nurse Practice, 7*(3), 48–54.

Brix, A. (1993). Critical thinking and theory-based practice. *Holistic Nurse Practice, 7*(3), 21–27.

Brown, H., Sorrell, J. (1993). Use of clinical journals to enhance critical thinking. *Nurse Educator, 18*(5), 16–18.

Bucher, L. (1993). The effects of imagery abilities and mental rehearsal on learning a nursing skill. *Journal of Nursing Education, 32*(7), 318–324.

Burfitt, S., Greiner, D., Miers, L. (1993). Professional nurse caring as perceived by critically ill patients: A phenomenologic study. *American Journal of Critical Care, 2*(6), 489–499.

Capuano, T. (1995). Clinical pathways: Practical approaches, positive outcomes. *Nursing Management, 26*(1), 34–37.

Carpenito, L. (1997). *Nursing diagnosis: Application to clinical practice* (7th ed.). Philadelphia, PA: Lippincott.

Carr, P. (1993). Discharge planning: Beyond hospital walls. *American Journal of Nursing, 93*(8), 38–39.

Case Management Society of America. (1995). *Standards of practice for case management.* Little Rock, AR: Author.

Cohen, E.L. (1996). *Nursing case managment in the 21st century.* St. Louis, MO: Mosby.

Cohen, E.L. (1999). *The outcomes mandate: Case management in health care today.* St. Louis, MO: Mosby.

Conger, M., Mezza, I. (1996). Fostering critical thinking in nursing students in the clinical setting. *Nurse Educator, 21*(3), 11–15.

Cravener, P. (1997). Promoting active learning in large lecture classes. *Nurse Educator, 22*(3), 22–26.

Doessey, B., Dossey, L. (1998). Body-mind-spirit: Attending to holistic care. *American Journal of Nursing, 98*(8), 35–38.

Dracup, K., Bryan-Brown, C. (1994). The three R's: Reading, writing, and research. *American Journal of Critical Care, 3*(5), 329–330.

Eskreis, T. (1998). Seven common legal pitfalls in nursing. *American Journal of Nursing, 98*(4), 34–41.

Facione, N., Facione, P., Sanchez, C. (1994). Critical thinking disposition as a measure of competent clinical judgment: The development of the California Critical Thinking Disposition Inventory. *Journal of Nursing Education, 33*(8), 345–351.

Flagler, S., Loper-Powers, S., Spitzer, A. (1988). Clinical teaching is more than evaluation alone! *Journal of Nurisng Education, 27*(8), 342–348.

Fonteyn, M. (1998). *Thinking strategies for nursing practice.* Philadelphia, PA: Lippincott-Ravin.

Fonteyn, M. (1991). Implications of clinical reasoning studies for critical care nursing. *Focus, 18*(4), 322–327.

Gordon, M. (1987). *Nursing diagnosis: Process and application.* New York, NY: McGraw-Hill.

Gorin, S., Arnold, J. (1998). *Health promotion handbook.* St. Louis, MO: Mosby.

Gruca, J. (1994). Bug of the week: A personification teaching strategy. *Journal of Nursing Education, 33*(4), 153–154.

Haag-Heitman, B., Kramer, A. (1998). Creating a clinical practice development model. *American Journal of Nursing, 98*(8), 39–44.

Hoeman, S. (1996). *Rehabilitation nursing.* St. Louis, MO: Mosby–Year Book.

Hogstel, M. (1998). *Community resources for older adults.* St. Louis, MO: Mosby.

Iyer, P., Taptich, B., Bernnochi-Losey, D. (1995). *Nursing process and nursing diagnosis* (3rd ed.). Philadelphia, PA: W.B. Saunders.

Jenks, J. (1993). The pattern of personal knowing in nurse clinical decision making. *Journal of Nursing Education, 32*(9), 399–405.

Johnson, M., Maas, M. (1997). *Nursing outcomes classification.* St. Louis, MO: Mosby.

Katooka-Yahiro, M., Saylor, C. (1994). A critical thinking model for nursing judgment. *Journal of Nursing Education, 33*(8), 351–356.

Kenney, E. (1998). Creating fulfilment in today's workplace: A guide for nurses. *American Journal of Nursing, 98*(5), 44–48.

Kramer, M. (1993). Concept clarification and critical thinking: Integrated processes. *Journal of Nursing Education, 32*(9), 387.

Kurfiss, J. (1988). *Critical thinking: Theory, research, practice, and possibilities.* ASHE-ERIC Higher Education Report No. 2. Washington, DC: Association for the Study of Higher Education.

Lashley, M., Wittstadt, R. (1993). Writing across the curriculum: An integrated curricular approach to developing critical thinking through writing. *Journal of Nursing Education, 32*(9), 422–424.

Loving, G. (1993). Competence validation and cognitive flexibility: A theoretical model grounded in nursing education. *Journal of Nursing Education, 32*(9), 387.

Manion, J. (1995). Understanding the seven stages of change. *American Journal of Nursing, 95*(4), 41–43.

Miller, M., Babcock, D. (1996). *Critical thinking applied to nursing.* St. Louis, MO: Mosby–Times Mirror.

Miller, M., Malcolm, N. (1990). Critical thinking in

the nursing curriculum. *Nursing and Health Care,* *11*(2), 67–73.

National League for Nursing. (1991). *Criteria for the evaluation of baccalaureate and higher degree programs in nursing* (6th ed.). New York, NY: Author.

National League for Nursing. (1990). *Educational outcomes of associate degree nursing programs: Roles and competencies.* New York, NY: Author.

National League for Nursing. (1989). *Role and competencies of graduates of diploma programs in nursing.* New York, NY: Author.

Norman, G. (1988). Problem-solving skills, solving problems, and problem-based learning. *Medical Education, 22,* 279–286.

North American Nursing Diagnosis Association. (1997). *Nursing diagnoses: Definitions and classifications.* Philadelphia, PA: Author.

Parrinello, K. (1995). Advanced practice nursing: An administrative perspective. *Critical Care Nursing Clinics of North America, 7*(1), 9–16.

Pesut, D., Herman, J. (1992). Metacognitive skills in diagnostic reasoning: Making the implicit explicit. *Nursing Diagnosis, 3*(4), 148–153.

Pless, B., Clayton, G. (1993). Clarifying the concept of critical thinking in nursing. *Journal of Nursing Education, 32*(9), 387.

Pond, E., Bradshaw, M., Turner, S. (1991). Teaching strategies for clinical thinking. *Nurse Educator, 16*(6), 18–22.

Rager, P. (1998). Emotional intelligence and the management edge. *Nursing Spectrum (FL ED), 8*(3), 3.

Reilly, D. (Ed.). (1978). *Teaching and evaluating the affective domain in nursing programs.* Thorofare, NJ: Charles B. Slack.

Rittman, M., Nedonma, N., Quesenberry, L., et al. (1993). Learning from "never again" stories. *American Journal of Nursing, 93*(6), 40–43.

Saarmann, L., Freitas, L., Rapps, J., Riegel, B. (1992). The relationship of education to critical thinking ability and values among nurses: Socialization into professional nursing. *Journal of Professional Nursing, 8*(1), 26–34.

Schoessler, M., Conedera, F., Bell, L., et al. (1993). Use of the Myers-Briggs type indicator to develop a continuing education department. *Journal of Nursing Staff Development, 9*(1), 8–13.

Siefker, J., Garrett, M., Van Genderen, A., Weis, M. (1998). *Fundamentals of case management.* St. Louis, MO: Mosby.

Tanner, C. (1993). More about critical thinking and clinical decision making. *Journal of Nursing Education, 32*(9), 387.

Tanner, C. (1993). Thinking about critical thinking. *Journal of Nursing Education, 32*(9), 99–100.

Tanner, C. (1983). Research on clinical judgment. In W.L. Holzemer (Ed.), *Review of research in nursing education* (pp. 1–32). Thorofare, NJ: Charles B. Slack.

Tanner, C., Benner, P., Chesla, C., Gordon, D. (1993). The phenomenology of knowing the patient. *Image, 25*(4), 273–280.

Taylor, C., Lillis, C., Lamone, P. (1997). *Fundamentals of nursing: The art and science of nursing care* (3rd ed.). Philadelphia, PA: J.B. Lippincott.

Toliver, J. (1988). Inductive reasoning: Critical thinking skills for clinical competence. *Clinical Nurse Specialist, 2*(4), 174–179.

Tschikota, S. (1993). The clinical decision-making processes of student nurses. *Journal of Nursing Education, 32*(9), 387.

Vaca, K., Vaca, B., Daake, C. (1998). Review of nursing home regulations. *MEDSURG NURSING, 7*(3), 165–171.

Valiga, T. (1983). Cognitive development: A critical component of baccalaureate nursing education. *Image, 15,* 115–119.

Wilkinson, J. (1996). *Nursing process: A critical thinking approach* (2nd ed.). Menlo Park, CA: Addison-Wesley.

Wolf, Z., Brennan, R., Ferchau, L., Magee, M., et al. (1997). Creating and implementing guidelines on caring for difficult patients: A research utilization project. *MEDSURG NURSING, 6*(3), 137–147.

Wolfe, Z. (1994). *Medication errors: The nursing experience.* Albany, NY: Delmar Publishers.

Culture and Diversity

American Nurses Association. (1991). *Position statement on cultural diversity in nursing practice.* Kansas City, MO: Author.

Campion, C. (1998). Embracing our differences. *Nursing Spectrum FL Ed., 8*(14), 5–6.

Geissler, E. (1999). *Pocket guide to cultural assessment* (2nd ed.). St. Louis, MO: Mosby.

Lester, N. (1998). Cultural competence: A nursing dialogue. *American Journal of Nursing, 98*(8), 26–34.

Lipson, J., Dibble, S., Minarik, P. (Eds.). (1996). *Culture and nursing care: A pocket guide.* San Francisco, CA: UCSF School of Nursing.

Salipante, D. (1998). Refusal of blood by a critically ill patient: A healthcare challenge. *Critical Care Nurse, 18*(2), 68–76.

General Critical Thinking

Barnes, C., McCabe, N. (1992). *Critical thinking: Educational imperatives.* San Francisco, CA: Jossey-Bass.

Block, P. (1996). *Stewardship: Choosing service over self-interest.* San Francisco, CA: Berrett-Koehler.

Boud, D., Feletti, G. (1991). *The challenge of problem based learning.* New York, NY: St Martins Press.

Brookfield. S. (1987). *Developing critical thinkers.* San Francisco, CA: Jossey-Bass.

Buzan, T. (1991). *Use both sides of your brain.* New York, NY: Fawcett Columbin.

Covey, S. (1989). *The seven habits of highly effective people.*® New York, NY: Simon & Schuster.

de Bono, E. (1985). *Six thinking hats: The power of focused thinking.* Boston: Little, Brown.

Eicher, J. (1996). Cognitive management™: Managing your organization's mind. *Performance Improvement, 35*(7), 12–15.

Ennis, R. (1990). Experience, education, and nurses' ability to make clinical judgments. *Nursing and Health Care, 11*(6), 290–294.

Ennis, R. (1987). A taxonomy of critical thinking dispositions and abilities. In J.B. Baron, J.J. Sternberg (Eds.), *Teaching thinking skills: Theory and practice.* New York, NY: Freeman.

Ennis, R., Millman, J., Tomoko, T. (1985). *Cornell critical thinking tests level X and level Z manual* (3rd ed.). Pacific Grove, CA: Midwest Publications.

Facione, P. (1992). *The California critical thinking skills test forms A and B.* Milbrae, CA: California Academic Press.

Facione, P. (1990). The APA report on critical thinking: A statement of expert consensus for purposes of educational assessment and instruction. In *ERIC Document Number 315 423.* Education and Research Information Center.

Facione, P.A., Facione, N.C. (1992). *The California critical thinking disposition inventory (CCTD)* and the *CCTDI test manual.* Milbrae, CA: California Academic Press.

Gardner, H. (1993). *Multiple intelligences.* New York, NY: Basic Books.

Goleman, D. (1995). *Emotional intelligence.* New York, NY: Bantam Books.

Halpern, D. (1984). *Thought and knowledge.* Hillsdale, NJ: Lawrence Erlbaum Associates.

Lehmkhul, D., Lamping, D. (1993). *Organizing for the creative person.* New York, NY: Crown Publishers, Inc.

Leiberstein, S. (1979). *Who owns what is in your head?* New York, NY: Hawthorn.

McPeck, J. (1981). *Critical thinking and education.* New York, NY: St. Martin's.

Meyers, C. (1986). *Teaching students to think critically.* San Francisco, CA: Jossey-Bass.

Paul, R. (1995). *Critical thinking: How to prepare students for a rapidly changing world.* Santa Rosa, CA: Foundation for Critical Thinking.

Paul, R. (1992). Critical thinking: What, why, and how? In C. Barnes (Ed.), *Critical thinking, an educational imperative.* San Francisco, CA: Jossey-Bass.

Paul, R., Binker, A. (Eds.). (1990). *Critical thinking: What every person needs to survive in a rapidly changing world.* Rohner Park, CA: Foundation for Critical Thinking and Moral Development.

Ruggiero, V. (1991). *The art of thinking: A guide to critical and creative thought* (3rd ed). New York, NY: HarperCollins.

Ruggiero, V. (1988). *Teaching thinking across the curriculum.* New York, NY: Harper & Row.

Senge, P. (1990). *The fifth discipline.* New York, NY: Doubleday.

Von Oech, R. (1983). *A whack on the side of the head: How you can be more creative.* New York, NY: Warner Books.

Wailey D. (1995). *Empires of the mind: Lessons to lead and succeed in a knowledge based world.* New York, NY: William Morrow and Co.

Watson, G., Glaser, E. (1980). *Watson-Glaser critical thinking appraisal manual.* Cleveland, OH: Psychological Corporation.

Weisinger, H. (1998). *Emotional intelligence at work.* San Francisco, CA: Jossey-Bass.

Moral and Ethical Reasoning

American Association of Critical Care Nurses. (1998). *Discovering your beliefs about healthcare choices (facilitator training manual): A guide to living wills and medical powers of attorney.* Aliso Viejo, CA: Author.

American Nurses Association. (1988). *Ethics in nursing: Position statements and guidelines.* Kansas City, MO: Author.

American Nurses Association. (1985). *Code for nurses with interpretive statements.* Kansas City, MO: Author.

Australian Nursing Council Inc. (1993). *Code of Ethics for Australian Nurses.* Canberra, Australia: Author.

Brock, M., Shank, M., Schellhause, E., Bruening, W. (1995). Teaching ethics to nurses. *Journal of Nursing Staff Development, 11*(5), 271–274.

Canadian Nurses Association. (1985). *Ethics code for nurses.* Ottawa, Canada: Author.

Chally, P. (1997). Nursing ethics. In K.K. Chitty (Ed.), *Professional nursing concepts and challenges* (2nd ed.). Philadelphia, PA: W.B. Saunders, pp. 363–384.

Chally, P., Loriz, L. (1998). Ethics in the trenches: Decision making in practice. *American Journal of Nursing, 98*(6), 17–20.

Curtin, L. (1978). A proposed model for critical ethical analysis. *Nursing Forum, 17,* 14.

De Wolf Bosek, M. (1995). Disregarding a physician's order: Insurrection or compassion? *MEDSURG Nursing, 4*(5), 396–397, 400.

De Wolf Bosek, M. (1995). Doing good: An ethical quandary. *MEDSURG Nursing, 4*(2), 154–156.

Foster, P. (1993). Helping students learn to make ethical decisions. *Holistic Nurse Practice, 7*(3), 28–35.

Gaul, A. (1995). Care: An ethical foundation for critical care nursing. *Critical Care Nurse, 6*(3) 134–135.

Haynor, P. (1998). Meeting the challenge of advance directives. *American Journal of Nursing, 98*(3), 26–32.

Jameton, A. (1984). *Nursing practice: The ethical issues.* Englewood Cliffs, NJ: Prentice Hall.

Johnstone, M. (1999). *Bioethics: A nursing perspective* (3rd ed.). Sydney, Australia: W.B. Saunders/Bailliere Tindall.

Johnstone, M. (1994). *Nursing and the injustices of the law.* Sydney, Australia: W.B. Saunders/Bailliere Tindall.

Kapala, B. (1997). Ethics. In J.M. Black, E. Matassarin-Jacobs (Eds.), *Medical-surgical nursing: Clinical management for continuity of care* (5th ed.). Philadelphia, PA: W.B. Saunders.

Kohlberg, L. (1976). Moral stages and moralization: The cognitive-developmental approach. In T. Likona (Ed.), *Moral development and behavior: Theory, research, and social issues* (pp. 34–35). New York, NY: Holt, Rinehart, & Winston.

Levenson, J., Pettrey, L. (1994). Controversial decisions regarding treatment and DNR: An algorithmic guide for the uncertain in decision-making ethics. (GUIDE). *American Journal of Critical Care, 3*(2), 87–91.

Paxman, G. (1993). Legal consult. *Nursing Spectrum (PA ED), 2*(20), 3.

Zimbelmann, J. (1994). Good life, good death, and the right to die: Ethical considerations for decisions at the end of life. *Journal of Professional Nursing, 10*(1), 22–37.

Nursing Research and Quality Improvement

Barrett, M. (1992). Optimizing nursing information systems. *Journal of Nursing Administration, 22*(10), 60–67.

Burns, N., Groves, S. (1997). *The practice of nursing research: Conduct, critique, and utilization* (3rd ed.). Philadelphia, PA: W.B. Saunders.

Dickenson-Hazard, N.N. (1995). Management perspectives. *Nursing Spectrum, 4*(7), 5.

Goode, C., Lovett, M., Hayes, J., Butcher, L. (1997). Use of research based knowledge in clinical practice. *Journal of Nursing Administration, 17*(12), 11–17.

Johnson, J.M., Reineck, C., Daigle-Bjerke, A., et al. (1995). Understanding research articles. *Journal of Nursing Staff Development, 11*(2), 95–99.

Joint Commission on the Accreditation of Healthcare Organizations. (1997). *Accreditation manual for hospitals.* Oakbrook Terrace, IL: Author.

Joint Commission on the Accreditation of Healthcare Organizations. (1990). *Primer on indicator development and application: Measuring quality in healthcare.* Oakbrook Terrace, IL: Author.

Joint Commission on the Accreditation of Healthcare Organizations. (1989). Characteristics of clinical indicators. *Quality Review Bulletin, 15*(11), 330–339.

Podogmy, K. (1991). Developing nursing-focused quality indicators: A professional challenge. *Journal of Nursing Care Quality, 6*(1), 47–52.

Polit, D., Hungler, B. (1999). *Nursing research* (6th ed.). Philadelphia, PA: Lippincott-Raven.

Remmlinger, E., Ault, S., Hanrahan, L. (1995). Information technology implications of case management. *Healthcare Information Management, 9*(1), 21–28.

Schnoor, E. (1997). Quality indicators and outcomes—so what? *Academy of Medical-Surgical Nurses News, 6*(5), 5.

Todd, W., Nash, D. (Eds.). (1997). *Disease management: A systems approach to improving patient outcomes.* St. Louis, MO: Mosby.

Wagner, P. (1995). Guide to identifying, collecting, and managing data. In J. Schmele (Ed.), *Quality management in nursing and health care* (pp. 410–418). Albany, NY: Delmar.

Williams. A. (1991). Development and application of clinical indicators for nursing. *Journal of Nurisng Care Quality, 6*(1), 1–5.

Teaching, Learning, and Test Taking

Berry, R. (1993). Effective patient education, part 1: Teaching adults. *Nursing Spectrum (PA ED), 2*(23), 14–16.

Berry, R. (1993). Effective patient education, part 2: Teaching children. *Nursing Spectrum (PA ED), 2*(24), 14–15.

Bloom, B. (Ed.). (1956). *Taxonomy of educational objectives. Handbook 1, Cognitive domain.* New York, NY: McKay.

Dickensen-Hazard, N. (1990). The psychology of successful test taking. *Pediatric Nursing, 16,* 66–67.

Dickensen-Hazard, N. (1989). Anatomy of a test question. *Pediatric Nursing, 15,* 480–481.

Dickensen-Hazard, N. (1989). Making the grade as a test taker. *Pediatric Nursing, 15,* 302–304.

Dunn, R. (1996). How learning style changes over a period of time. *InterEd* (Special Edition), January, pp. 3–4.

Katz, J. (1997). Providing effective patient teaching. *American Journal of Nursing, 97*(5), 33–36.

Keane, M. (1993). Preferred learning styles and study strategies in a linguistically diverse baccalaureate nursing student population. *Journal of Nursing Education, 32*(5), 215–221.

Kintgen-Andrews, J. (1991). Critical thinking and nursing education: Perplexities and insights. *Journal of Nursing Education, 30*(4), 152–157.

Klaassens, E. (1988). Improving teaching for thinking. *Nurse Educator, 13*(6), 15–19.

Kolb, D. (1976). *Learning style inventory: Self-scoring test and interpretation booklet.* Boston, MA: McBer & Co.

Komelasky, A., Bond, B. (1993). The effect of two forms of learning reinforcement upon parental retention of CPR skills. *Pediatric Nursing, 19*(1), 77, 96–98.

Meltzer, M., Palau, S.M. (1997). *Learning strategies in nursing: Reading, studying, and test taking* (2nd ed.). Philadelphia, PA: W.B. Saunders.

Mollan-Masters, R. (1992). *You are smarter than you think.* Ashland, OR: Reality Productions.

Nugent, P., Vitale, B. (1997). *Test success: Test-taking techniques for beginning nursing student* (2nd ed.). Philadelphia, PA: F.A. Davis.

Ouellette, F. (1988). A textbook coding tool, part 1: Assessing elements that promote analytic abilities. *Nurse Educator, 13*(5), 8–13.

Robinson, A. (1993). *What smart students know: Maximum grades, optimum learning, minimum time.* New York, NY: Crown Trade Paperbacks.

Sides, M., Korchek, N. (1997). *Nurses guide to successful test-taking* (3rd ed.). Philadelphia, PA: J.B. Lippincott.

Index

Note: Page numbers in *italics* refer to illustrations; page numbers followed by t refer to tables.